Force 46
Strength
and
Conditioning

The John Stucky Perspective

Transformative Knowledge for Fitness
and Physical Education Design

Anthony Tridico

PAGE PUBLISHING
Conneaut Lake, PA

First originally published by Page Publishing 2023

ISBN 979-8-88793-785-4 (pbk)
ISBN 979-8-88793-796-0 (digital)

Printed in the United States of America

Preface

As you will see after reading this book, the ideas and echo chambers of the concepts of fitness, training and exercise modes and methods can be broken down to individual proprietary interests that create many myths, fallacies, and confusing perceptions that lead to cultural problems in the study of human movement and how you can take the best care of your body for a lifetime. By nature, the echo chambers in all aspects of fitness and education create confused knowledge bases with many shortcomings, and the proverbial circle jerk, that is the echo chamber, becomes a theory guided by self-promotion and deceit both knowingly and unknowingly.

You cannot address physical education design without addressing the political and corruptive practices that are rampant/prevalent in public education (kindergarten through college) as well as the cultural problems with coaching (in any sport). All these ties with real science and art to address the ills society creates in all facets of problem-solving for the greater good in any given area. The one person who was far advanced in all aspects of training and personified excellence as a human being was Coach Stucky.

I have observed many alarming trends in sports training and fitness information, as well as alarming trends in physical education over the last thirty years. Social media is saturated with training information and opinion, which reaches all aspects of society. This is especially alarming and often detrimental to the multisport athlete at the lower levels (e.g., kindergarten through high school). Siff made the statement that other than periodization, no other Russian sporting secret has captured the attention of Western coaches and athletes as powerfully as so-called plyometrics (Siff, 2003). I have observed two other training concepts that should be added to this list and, to this day, are regarded as the magic bullet of success. The two other training concepts are specialization and sport-specific training. These two concepts have been so misrepresented with the lower levels of sport and specifically with the multisport athlete. Misrepresentation of these concepts has led to crazy belief systems that are as ingrained in our society as the cardiovascular doctrine from the 1960s. The misrepresentation or misinterpretation of all of these concepts has had a negative impact on the multisport athlete as well as the importance of physical education.

Tribute to John Stucky

"I knew when I left the weight room at the University of Arkansas for the final time that all people should learn to train like this!"

Coach Stucky was a pioneer in strength and conditioning for athletes. If Coach Stucky wasn't the first true strength and conditioning coach, then he is as close to being the first as they come. In 1970, Coach Stucky began a successful two-year stint playing in the CFL for the British Columbia Lions. His interest in coaching and sharing strength training with other football players, however, drew him back to Kansas State. While earning a master's degree in physical education, Coach Stucky was a freshman-line coach and ran the Kansas State strength and conditioning program. In 1974, Coach Stucky went to Wichita State where he was both the defensive line coach and strength coach. In 1977, Coach Stucky moved to the University of Arkansas where he served as strength coach and linebacker coach. During this time, the Razorbacks appeared in the Orange Bowl, Fiesta Bowl, and Sugar Bowl. In 1980, Coach Stucky moved to North Carolina State University and served as a defensive line and strength coach. He was able to give up his on-field coaching responsibilities and run the growing strength and conditioning program full-time. In 1984, Coach Stucky went to Oklahoma State as a full-time strength coach. He spent four seasons running the weight room there and worked with athletes Thurman Thomas and Barry Sanders. On his strength program, Coach Stucky commented, "We're not preparing a guy to be a bodybuilder. We're preparing him to be a running, jumping, explosive athlete." Coach Stucky returned to Arkansas once again in 1988 to take charge of the Razorbacks' strength and conditioning program. Under his guidance, the Razorbacks won back-to-back Southwest Conference championships in 1988 and 1989. (Coach Stucky also coached Barry Foster who is another great running back.) Coach Stucky had earned about every major accolade that can be bestowed on a strength and conditioning professional (e.g., in spring 2001, Coach Stucky was named one of the ten master strength and conditioning coaches by the Collegiate Strength and Conditioning Coaches Association—the title was the highest honor that could be achieved as a strength and conditioning coach; under Coach Stucky's leadership, the Vols compiled an 80–16 record and won the national title in 1998; the Vols also captured two Southeastern Conference crowns and three Eastern Division titles in the eight year span; Coach also was the strength and conditioning coach for the Arkansas basketball team that won the national title in 1994 and went to three final fours, which I witnessed firsthand because we often trained together in the weight room at the University of Arkansas; Coach Stucky was also named national coach of the year in 1996 by the Professional Football Strength and Conditioning Coaches Association; and Coach Stucky was also twice picked by his SEC peers as the league's top strength coach), and yet, having personally gone through his workouts for years, he was even greater than the accolades he earned.

Coach Stucky was a quiet, calm man who carried himself in a physical and humble manner! You visibly understood that you were standing next to a legend, and yet those words would never come out of his mouth. He was just happy to look forward to the lifts of the day and watch people get better. I have earned many accomplishments and awards over the last thirty years. The best compliment I ever received, and hang on to like it was yesterday, was when an assistant strength coach pulled me aside and said, "Coach Stucky paid you a compliment!"

I was totally lost in a surreal moment and looked confused and excited at the same time and responded, "What did Coach say?"

The assistant strength coach replied, "Coach Stucky said he had never seen anyone improve as much as you!"

To this day, that set my life's course and continued the quest for expertise. I went on to Boise State University, and Joe Kenn immediately took me in as an assistant coach (because he knew Coach Stucky's reputation) and put me to work coaching immediately and even put my name tag on the door. I gained a lot of knowledge with Coach Kenn and being a graduate student at Boise State University in the exercise and sports studies program.

My father passed away in 1996 while I was at Boise State University, so I decided to move back to Pennsylvania and teach and coach in the public schools. This decision was also directly related to my experience back at Arkansas when our football coach was fired. Arkansas made a poor choice in who they hired, and this sorry excuse for a coach had a long-standing issue with Coach Stucky. I did not know this at the time. The only thing I knew was this so-called football coach came into a legend's weight room and said that all players have to squat with safety squat bars, not regular barbells, and tried to play backdoor politics behind the scenes. This fact was inconceivable to me, and yet it happened.

Coach Stucky had no time for this kind of unprofessional incompetence, and long story short, Coach leaves the University of Arkansas to take the head strength and conditioning position at the University of Tennessee. I remember that the teammates I was speaking with at that moment were all happy for Coach Stucky, but I distinctly remember saying that Arkansas will get worse quickly, and that was exactly what happened. The other thing my teammates said was that Coach Stucky said he will win the national title at Tennessee within three years. The University of Tennessee did exactly that, winning the national championship game against Florida State University in 1998!

The fact that I witnessed firsthand the absurd politics at the division I level (i.e., that you could be the best strength coach in the country, and if the football coach gets fired, the new football coach can bring his own coach in, and you can be replaced for no reason at all). This was where I was so disgusted, that I realized that I likely did not want that lifestyle and felt I could greatly help many kids and adults in public schools without the petty money/ego-driven ignorance at the university level. Ironically, over the course of twenty five years, I found out that human ignorance is alive and well in all aspects of public schools or likely in any job that is part of a system in general. The only true way to get away from that nonsense is to be self-employed and run your own business, which I currently do now, or shrug your shoulders and not make waves, just be status quo.

The other driving motivator Coach Stucky personified was the love for the kids and his quest for being a Christian. He loved to help people to learn to honor the Lord. He wanted people to have something more, which, in short, was eternal life. I have yet to reach that level of appreciation for his profound faith, but this was just another prime example why Coach Stucky was at the top of the mountain in strength and conditioning and in faith. The rest of us will always have to look up and hope we can keep getting better.

Coach Stucky coached many famous athletes like Peyton Manning, Barry Sanders, Thurman Thomas, Quinn Grovey, Corliss Williamson, and most importantly, Coach Stucky coached me! The knowledge I gained can't be found simply in a book or in a scientific laboratory. I am very proud that I am just an extension of the man, and that realization helped me understand that it is not relevant how good you are individually, it is only important that you realize that it is what other people/God did for you that makes you great. (This statement is likely not understood in the professional bureaucracy that has now overtaken college sports and trickled down to the high schools and middle schools.) Coach Stucky would not be pleased with the changes in sports currently coming out of the COVID-19 years. Coach Stucky was not a get-back coach that you see on ESPN, ABC, and CBS prime-time games that make the college strength coach look like a fool! Coach Stucky was never subservient to political titles and the money! Coach Stucky was a servant to his faith and his love for his kids and family. To this day, Coach Stucky's gifts that I was able to take have allowed me to be great in my own way, and I could not have gotten there if it wasn't for him.

After all the schooling—all the research of Russian manuals and reading and dissecting anything I could get my hands on, all the state level presentations and self-driven professional development with other great coaches along the way—I have come full circle, and my program design process and philosophy comes right back to Coach Stucky along with the exact feeling I had back in 1992 that every human being should train like this!

Knowledge versus Perception/Opinion

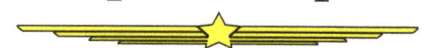

I heard Louie Simmons speak, many years ago, on two different occasions at the Pennsylvania state strength and conditioning conference. A person who wants to continually get better should hope to glean a few pieces of very important information that maybe they forgot about or just weren't aware of. These few pieces of information can really help for continual improvement and lead to application of knowledge that has not been duplicated in a science lab. The idea of following science has never been more abused than with the COVID-19 epidemic and with the No Child Left Behind Act in the early 2000s. Both these issues have led society into complete disarray, ignorant echo chambers, and political corruption.

Science is very important, however, I have observed that the great practitioners in weight lifting and strength and conditioning are always far ahead of "science." The reason for this is that when a great practitioner is working with twenty-seven men and women's sports, and lifts are prescribed in certain sequences, it is nearly impossible to recreate that environment in a controlled laboratory environment. A second reason for this gap between science and practice (i.e., *art*) is the nature of the United States' culture to self-promote or push self-serving agendas over real knowledge and practical application as I will outline throughout the book.

There are endless examples of self-proclaimed titles in the fitness industry. The list actually is endless on the next magic bullet that was never correct to begin with. However, I chose the following studies to be some of the prime examples of nonsense that become published junk science. The junk science then becomes a new echo chamber yet at the same time is the same rehash of old trash that leads to poor coaching, poor physical education, poor weight loss claims, and poor certifications that allow misguided fitness fanatics the belief systems that confound any sense of reality or truth. I laugh at the newfound terms in training (e.g., HIIT—high-intensity interval training, MICT—moderate-intensity cardiorespiratory training), and somehow, these new-wave terms signify different training versus weight training, warped perceptions like doing yoga is a better form of fitness for nonathletes, walking on a treadmill is better fitness later in life, buying a Peloton bike for $1,500–$2,500 for fitness, walking ten thousand steps for fitness, targeting heart rate and circuit training are key for training, BMI (body mass index) is the standard for identifying obesity, long slow distance running is best for conditioning, etc.—all these echo chambers will be given a reality check throughout this book.

As you will see after reading this book, I always believed and it has proven to be true for more than thirty years and many thousands of athletes and clients that there really should only be one term to describe great training, and that term is *strength and conditioning*. Coach Stucky was way ahead of his time, and there has never been a time where the need to have that kind of knowledge to be present in the corrupt Wild West times that society is currently in. If the transformational knowledge Coach Stucky possessed is not promoted, then the misguided echo chambers will continue the rampant ignorance that we see, and real strength and conditioning will be lost forever. This book's intention is to set the record on the reality of what great training should be for all humans in a no-nonsense fashion (i.e., the Coach Stucky way)!

The first study I ran across recently on Google News was titled "Yet 'Another' Study Finds that Regular Training Builds Muscle Strength." This latest study was published in the *Scandinavian*

Journal of Medicine & Science in Sports. The take-home claim from this study is why working out less intensely is a smart move. As you will see as you read my book, if one reads and understands the science I have researched as well as my own personal strength and conditioning experience of actually lifting, then the statement the article in question is promoting is far from the truth or any sense of reality.

Researchers out of Japan and Australia recruited thirty-six healthy young adults for this study. They were curious to see how doing the same workout—an arm resistance exercise lowering a heavy dumbbell in a bicep curl—at different intensities and frequencies affected fitness results. One group did a set of six contractions one day a week (low intensity, low frequency), another did a set of 30 contractions one day a week (high intensity, low frequency), and the last did a set of six contractions five days a week (low intensity, high frequency). The study states that everyone kept up with this routine for four weeks before getting their muscle strength and muscle thickness measured. After the month was up, those in the group who did a set of six contractions five times a week were the only ones who saw significant gains in both muscle strength and thickness. The group who did 30 contractions in one day saw an increase in thickness but not strength, while the group who did six contractions in one day did not increase muscle size or strength. This study demonstrates that if muscle strength and thickness are your goals (and they should be, as they've been associated with things like weight management, heart health, and blood sugar balance), you'll want to do lighter, shorter workouts—but do them more frequently. (Loewe 2022)

The article then added the section "What It Means for You."

Consider this yet another reason to opt for frequent repetitions of Zone 2 exercise (the level of exercise where you can still hold a conversation) over the occasional all-out workout. "People think they have to do a lengthy session of resistance training in the gym, but that's not the case. Just lowering a heavy dumbbell slowly once or six times a day is enough," study author—Ken Nosaka, PhD—says in a statement. "We only used the bicep curl exercise in this study, but we believe this would be the case for other muscles also, at least to some extent." (In MindBodyGreen's MBG moves library, there is a treasure trove of lower-impact routines tailored to each muscle group.) MindBodyGreen states that pairing these resistance moves with plenty of walking and standing throughout the day for an exercise routine that's effective and sustainable over the long run. As far as how much time to spend exercising a week, one 2018 study found the "Goldilocks zone" of physical activity was at least 150 minutes of moderately intense aerobic exercise a week. (Loewe 2022)

Nosaka and his coauthors note those who opt for less intense workout routines still need to carve out time to rest and recover. "Be sure to stay hydrated, keep up with static stretching, and potentially invest in a foam roller or massage gun." Taking a turmeric supplement can also help your muscles fully recover between frequent workouts. The full-spectrum turmeric in MBG's turmeric potency+, for example, has been clinically researched and shown to reduce muscle soreness and improve strength between exercise sessions. (Loewe 2022)

The takeaway

Want to get stronger but not a fan of high-intensity training? Don't sweat it. As Nosaka says (and his new research supports): "If you're just going to the gym once a week, it's not as effective as doing a bit of exercise every day at home."

As you read the book, you will see that there are many different types of strength that is needed in all programs along with many different types of muscular tension. Differing levels of intensity throughout the week along with compound multijointed lifts are necessary. Fast, slow, eccentric, along with differing rep ranges and rest between sets are all part of a relevant program. Most of the research article doesn't even identify the type of strength the study actually slightly addresses. In this study, lowering a weight slowly means eccentric strength emphasis, so the PhD who authored this article needs to state that and not just say strength. You should understand this by the time you read this book. A huge limitation to this study is why would you even study a group of people who lift six repetitions one day per week? Talk about wasting your time. The fact that we are researching a bicep curl is even more silly, which, again, is why lab studies are so difficult. Most studies try to create the simplest design to reach a desired conclusion, but the design is so irrelevant that the very conclusion that is gained is nothing but irrelevant information. Yet most people will read this study and lay claim that this is good training.

A second study from this same group of researchers at Edith Cowan University (ECU) and also published in the *European Journal of Applied Physiology* reinforces their same belief system that those who just lower weights can achieve the same results as those who both lift and lower them despite only doing half the apparent work. This echo chamber of education is pushing the scientific belief that low rep but regular eccentric or lengthening muscle contraction as opposed to concentric or isometric (i.e., lifting a weight and holding a weight) respectively is the best way to increase muscle strength and size. The fascination of size of muscle over actual training for health factors (e.g., blood pressure, weight loss, dynamic flexibility, injury prevention, sport performance, etc.) is the same nonsense that BMI and the cardiovascular doctrine have helped create the endless myths and uneducated self-promotion for sport coaches, personal trainers, physical educators, and the fitness industry in general. This snake oil and poor educational inquiry can only be tamed if people can learn to be able to dissect research and stop reading the headlines and taking the headline as scientific fact.

This study consisted of one group of just eccentric lowering, one group of just lifting the dumbbells, and a third group of doing both. The fourth and final control group was tasked with doing nothing relatable. The mode was to perform dumbbell curls just twice a week over a five-week period. The results were pretty clear. While all groups attained some kind of benefit, Team Lift only saw improvement in their concentric strength. The other two groups (Team Lower and Team Both) improved in their concentric, eccentric, and isometric strength. "But while Team Both definitely did okay, Team Lower performed better by posttrial muscle thickness, boasting a 7.2 percent gain in swoleness versus Team Both's 5.4 percent increase. You'd be forgiven for feeling like this all sounds wildly counterintuitive. After all, we literally called strength training "lifting," and people in weight rooms generally tend to measure success by counting how many pounds they can push up into the air. According to this research, however, that might just be a waste of time" (Harrison 2022). As you should be able to see at this point, a person must be able to dissect research and not get lost in the title of the research to be able to read between the lines with actual comprehension.

Dr. Mel Siff did a great job addressing regimes of muscular work in his *Supertraining* book.

> For example, some researchers maintain
> that the largest strength gains are made with

dynamic (concentric) actions and others state the largest strength gains occur with isometric tension. Moreover, careful analysis of the experimental design reveals that similar contradictions are associated with invalid generalizations of results obtained in different laboratories, under unnatural conditions, on different muscle groups of subjects of different standards, using different loads and movement speeds. For instance, it was established that with maximal isometric tension of the biceps (elbow flexed to ninety degrees), subjects were able to develop a force 6.5–10.0 kg greater than the maximal weight that could be lifted concentrically. However, this changes with a decrease in load and an increase in speed of movement. The electrical activity in the biceps muscle while lifting a weight of 50–80 percent of maximum is significantly greater than it is during the period when it is subsequently held statically, both in magnitude and the production of strength. (Stepano and Burlakov 1963; Monogarov and Laputin 1966; Scheraev 1954, 1957; Rasch and Pierson 1960; Yanchevsky and Steklove 1966 in Siff 2003)

Thus, there is an important difference in the characteristics of the muscular force displayed depending upon the magnitude of the load and the speed of movement. It should be pointed out that the torque produced by the muscles increases approximately fourfold up to an angle of 90 degrees during elbow flexion. Therefore, if you compare the force of a maximal isometric action developed at an angle of 90 degrees and the maximum weight that can be raised from an angle of 180 degrees, then the force in the first case is greater. Consequently, if one is referring to the development of muscular strength, then to discuss superiority in the dynamic versus the isometric regime is scarcely appropriate because the biomechanical conditions for the production of strength are not comparable. If it is necessary to compare the training effect of a certain regime, then you must first establish which kind of strength is being measured. (Siff 2003)

A similar approach is necessary when comparing the advantages of eccentric and concentric muscular work. Bethe (1929) showed that the force a muscle develops with a maximal overcoming action (concentric strength) is between 1.2 and 1.6 times less than the resistance strength and contracting muscle displays when it is stretched (eccentric strength). Some examples of the superiority of eccentric strength over concentric strength for some muscle groups are as follows: 22 percent for the arms, 46.8 percent for the forearms, and 50 percent for the knee extensors. According to Semyonov's study of untrained subjects (1968), the maximal isometric force developed by the knee extensors at an angle of 120 degrees is 465 newtons and 401 newtons in the concentric regime. For combined regimes, the largest strength (504 newtons) was recorded for slow eccentric action exerted after preliminary maximal isometric tension (under conditions of equivalent forced-knee flexion using an electric motor to offer resistance) and 453 newtons produced for eccentric action exerted after preliminary concentric work. (Siff 2003)

Eccentric work uses significantly less energy than concentric work. It has been demonstrated by replacing concentric with eccentric actions that the expenditure of energy is almost halved when movement velocity does not exceed 0.12 metres/second (Chauveau 1904). These conclusions have been corroborated more recently. It has been revealed that more energy is expended by the concentric versus the isometric action of a muscle. The energy expenditure for muscle lengthening is also less than that for isometric action (Fenn 1924; Hartree and Hill 1928; Hill 1930; Cattle 1983). However, it should be emphasized that this advantage of eccentric work is displayed only with slow movements and large loads.

Therefore, there is no reason to associate these advantages with the potential to develop the ability for quick and powerful movements in concentric work. (Siff 2003)

This science from Siff shows that the idea of eccentric strength is clearly not new at all, and the great strength coaches have always been aware of its appropriateness. Coach Stucky clearly understood this, but again, eccentric work is just a tiny piece of the puzzle, and the fact that we have science being reported in the year 2022 that eccentric work is vastly superior to size and benefit as well as purporting that just doing lowering of random weights is proven to be all that you need to do and forget about concentric work is just another example of epic ignorance in fitness and training.

Siff (2003) also cited research that eccentric training has shown that significant levels of postexercise soreness (i.e., delayed onset muscle soreness) are produced after regimes of eccentric training. "The DOMS typically peaks after twenty-four to seventy-two hours after exercise and then disappears" (Friden et al. 1983). However, in reality, it appears that DOMS is much more prevalent in beginners, and experienced lifters often do not experience DOMS.

The problems from the way research has been conducted and promoted in the United States has led to many foolish belief systems, echo chambers, myths, very poor certification programs, and confusion among the general public. This study alone will allow the next middle school physical education teacher, hopelessly pathetic sports coach, and figurehead-status quo public school administrator to continue the ignorance that seems prevalent and well established in our current society with no end in sight. I do not want to take too much time outlining every sad flaw in the study because I think when you read the rest of this book, you will then realize how much of what the fitness industry and educational system is pumping is still the same snake oil it always has been and being an expert or informed consumer is becoming even more difficult, and our public schools are not helping but rather aiding in "drinking the Kool-Aid" and promoting the "snake oil" echo chambers in all aspects of education, expertise, and opinion. Our world could be better if people could "wipe the shit out of their eyes so they could see!" And the world would be better if we could hear Coach Stucky in person one more time!

The second study is titled "The Best Workout Routine Ever, According to Science!" As Brooks Kubik stated, "If anyone ever tries to sell you a book, course, or exercise machine based on "scientific" weight training principles, hit them hard and run like hell!" The article starts with "every so often new workout plans will move into the mainstream. For instance, in the 1980s, step aerobics were all the rage (this is sadly true). "In the 1990s, at-home workout tapes like Buns of Steel, Tae Bo, etc...were king. Then there were similar exercise trends in every decade that followed. However, there have always been some tried and true methods that can lead to an incredible physique and great health" (Richardson 2022). Bennett Richardson, DPT, PT, CSCS writes the article and outlines one of the best, simplest resistance training routines there is. With all the letters after his name, one would think you could conclude that the writer is very intelligent and experienced with strength and conditioning. As you will see, he speaks like the same echo chamber in education and fitness, and it is a far cry from the legend John Stucky or my training programs.

> The next heading in the article states, "Sets and Reps for the Optimal Workout." This workout consists of four exercises, ten reps per exercise, and three sets of each exercise for three sessions per week. All the exercises in this workout are multi-joint, compound movements. Because of this, each movement works tons of different muscles. "To get even more calorie burn, this workout routine is set up as a circuit" (Richardson 2022). A circuit is a type of workout in which one exercise is performed one after the other. "In this way, the muscles that are worked during the first exercise are able to rest while the next exercise is performed. You'll want to rest for as little as possible during this routine. This will help to increase the cardiorespiratory demands of the workout and will lead to incredible results" (Richardson 2022).

At this point, you might ask what is wrong with this article and title. Most people just look at the title, and if it sounds good and has the term *science*, then it must be true. This is completely untrue. The author was correct that compound lifts are better, but Coach Stucky knew this back in the 1970s minimally. How lifts are sequenced daily, what lifts, how heavy, slow, or fast, and how many reps, rest intervals, etc. are extremely important and rarely addressed properly in most research. Compound lifts for high reps and cardiovascular effect are simply fingernails worth of strength endurance, and that is it. It is not a magic training scheme. In fact, this training would lead to overtraining very quickly. The idea of doing front squats and dead lift in the same day is more of a bodybuilding lifting concept. Bodybuilding has nothing to do with human movement. The fact that it is 2022 and we are seeing articles written about promoting this as good training is scary in and of itself.

The author emphasized four compound lifts with ten reps. Ten reps is strength endurance that is simply a standard number. The four compound lifts are fine, but lifting the same four lifts at the same rep range and not identify individual deficiencies and needs in an actual program design is ridiculous. The outdated circuit concept, in addition, is truly sad because now the author wants to make sure you have little rest so your heart rate stays up. It seems like we can never get away from the cardiovascular doctrine no matter what, and that is part of the status quo in education as well. This is sloppy design at best because no top strength coach is going to do these compound lifts for cardio three days per week and claim that science proves it is best for anything. This totally misses all the science that is presented in this book.

One of the great things about Coach Stucky was he never fell into the ridiculous echo chambers, and his program design from back in the 1990s is more impressive and relevant today. As you will also see and hopefully comprehend as you read this book, categorizing human beings as athlete, nonathlete, toning, functional, core training, and all the other buzzwords really misses the boat, so read on!

These two studies are perfect examples of highly educated (probably good human beings) that are so off the mark of what great training and fitness is that it is a big reason why I felt it was time to write this book. I have experienced a lot of what people call being educated and that education leading to complete ignorance in reality. Echo chambers are created, and people spend huge money to go to college to be exposed to really improper knowledge. But since everyone is saying the same thing (knowledge wise) and passing it on as science, then the next group of deficient experts keep the rhetoric rolling down the same wrong path. I completed two master's degrees, one in exercise and sport studies and another in educational leadership (principal K-12). I completed my bachelor of science in kinesiology at the University of Arkansas. With all the knowledge that I studied and tested on, the real learning that made me know what I know today was actually lifting under a real strength and conditioning coach. That strength and conditioning coach was John Stucky.

A major issue with strength training is not identifying great lifts. A major issue is really program design on an annual plan and how that looks like and works on a daily and weekly basis along with ignoring all the junk science and snake oil claims. It is as much an art as it is science, and the science has to be the correct science, and identifying what is the correct science is difficult in and of itself. The other major strength and conditioning coach who helped advance my knowledge was Joe Kenn at Boise State University. Working for Joe was great, and working the floor specifically really gave me better insight to coaching and better training. Jerry Shreck, Todd Burkey, Jeremy Hoy, and Doug Smith were, and still are, great strength coaches whom I spent many years speaking with at conferences and talking shop. The certifications and all the other education really were way beneath and far less relevant to the expertise I currently have.

At one time, the CSCS was really the only recognized strength certification specifically for what we know as strength and conditioning coaches whom Coach Stucky was a pioneer. As time went on, many groups with their own echo chambers started to be included in the NSCA. You previously had all kinds of frivolous personal trainer certifications (which we still do) and then nutrition groups also entered the NSCA. It was easy to see that the NSCA had lost and strayed from its original message and intent. Just previous to me taking the Pennsylvania state director position with the NSCA, the college strength coaches had taken real issues on numerous chapters and guidelines with the NSCA, and they created the CSCCA certification for college strength coaches whom Coach Stucky was a leader in.

I was a college guy, but because I was a high school strength coach at the time, I was not allowed to take that test, which made me realize that there are real problems in training that are not going to get fixed. The certifications alone do not make an expert at this point, and like in all professions, some are really good in strength and conditioning and most are not. Coach Stucky was great and that set the tone to where Force 46 is today. The following algebraic equations in training are taken from the book *Supertraining Sixth Edition*. This little piece of science is very important to program design, and most people have never even seen this science.

Algebraic Relations and Training

Two algebraic laws may be applied to the interaction between different means, methods, and techniques in strength (and all sports) training, which are important because they are not generally obeyed in training.

The commutative law: $A*B = B*A$
The associative law: $A*(B*C) = (A*B)*C$

A system may be said to be commutative if it does not matter in which order the operations are done in that system. In sports training, this is not the case since the order in which one carries out exercises or kinds of exercises can change the outcome (i.e., clean*squat does not equal squat*clean).

The associative law is also relevant. A system is said to be associative if the operations follow this law: $A*(B*C) = (A*B)*C$. Sports training is nonassociative since the use of means A followed by a complex of two means B and C does not

> yield the same result as a complex of means A and B followed by the use of a single means C. Thus, the use of a muscle endurance regime A before a complex of plyometrics B and Olympic lifting C does not yield the same results as the use of a complex of muscle endurance A and plyometrics B followed by Olympic lifting C on its own (Siff 2003).

This mathematical science cited by Siff alone tells you that any physical therapist, personal trainer, or CSCS who writes articles about "The Best Workout Routine Ever, According to Science" should be understood as scientifically false and nothing but drinking the Kool-Aid and ignorance. You will see that Siff already criticized the West for basing training programs on simple anatomy many years ago, and yet the status quo education in the West is alive and well still promoting incorrect beliefs as expertise. Therefore, how a strength and conditioning coach structures the lifts and training is very important and often not even thought of by many today. This is where Coach Stucky was a pioneer and more relevant today than ever.

> In addition to volume, the structure of the training scheme is vitally important in every sport. Verkhoshanky (1997) stated that an issue that is also of real concern is the fact that classical computation of periodization training schemes generally utilizes only two factors in regulating the training of the athlete, namely the volume and intensity of the training load. This is one reason why the book *Supertraining* (Siff 2003) paid special attention to Matveyev's attempt to include technical skill training as one of the factors involved in periodization. (Siff 2003)

These ideas are equally important in creating a great physical education design and theory.

To our knowledge, my wife and I are the only physical educators in the country who deliberately pay attention to this information. Therefore, following the science is only half of the equation.

I have observed over the last thirty plus years the individuals who understand that the "art" element is the other half of the equation to true improvement in knowledge and ideas. Few and far between seem to grasp this understanding. The application of the art (i.e., skill) in training, teaching, and literally any other aspect of life is necessary to really further knowledge.

> The organization of training is as much a matter of art, trial and error, and intuition as it is of science. Therefore, periodization schemes can serve as approximate guidelines to be followed and modified by ongoing analysis of various physiological and psychological markers of progress. (Siff 2003)

If individuals only follow the science, then they will be the ones left behind. I took two specific pieces of knowledge from Louie Simmons that I thank him for every day. The first was "I encourage you all to read." Louie went after many so-called academic experts who did not share his knowledge because Louie did not receive his knowledge from a university. The second piece of information that I thank Louie for is his speaking to paying attention to the nervous system when designing programs. This played a big role in how I chose to write higher-level programs for accomplished lifters. Thank you, Louie, and of course, Coach Stucky!

George Hackenschmidt wrote a book titled *The Way to Live.* This book was originally published in 1908. It is clear the message had been ignored in the United States and especially when Dr. Cooper came along with highly incorrect and long-term corrupt cardiovascular doctrine. Hackenschmidt stated the following:

> It is a well-known fact that the majority of men today are relatively weak, whereas the strug-

gle for existence demands now more than at any previous epoch that we should all be strong! The reader may think that physical strength is not a necessity, but I will try and prove to him that man cannot derive real enjoyment from life unless he possesses a powerful and healthy physical constitution. I have come to the distinct conclusion that the physical constitution of the human frame never was intended merely for study but rather for manual and bodily exercise. I have found that those who have lived an active outdoor life have retained and enjoyed a brightness born of health far longer than others. A famous physician expressed himself as follows: "If I think of my experiences during a thirty years practice, I cannot recall many cases where a patient became ill through to great an exertion on his physical system, whereas I remember many hundreds who have contracted serious illness through mental strain and brain fog, and their complete recovery invariably was a slow and difficult process."

Hackenschmidt went on to say, "The most effective means of preventing all the disadvantages and evil consequences of a neglected exercise of body and muscles is methodical physical training." The fact that his expertise was back in 1908 and our country has missed this understanding by following the cardiovascular doctrine should raise a huge red flag to what is intelligence and what is best for humankind.

Brooks D. Kubik wrote a book called *Dinosaur Training: Lost Secrets of Strength and Development*. This book was published in 1996. I knew Brooks hit a home run on the very first page of his book. Kubik stated the following:

> I have studied the art of weight training for most of my life. By the way, as a brief aside, that's

exactly what productive weight training truly is: an ART…not a science. If anyone ever tries to sell you a book, course, or exercise machine based on "scientific" weight training principles, hit him hard and quick and run like hell!

Kubik has many prominent quotes from a wide variety of people with very telling statements. I would like to share a few of my favorites.

Ralph Waldo Emerson stated, "Society is always taken by surprise by any example of common sense."

Anatole France stated, "If fifty million people say a foolish thing, it is still a foolish thing."

George Hackenschmidt stated, "The knowledge of one's strength entails a real master over oneself; it breeds energy and courage, helps one over the most difficult tasks of life, and procures contentment and true enjoyment of living."

Victor Hugo stated, "There is one thing stronger than all the armies in the world, and that is an idea whose time has come."

Sir Winston Churchill stated, "Difficulties mastered are opportunities won."

G. K. Chesterton stated, "It isn't that they can't see the solution. It is that they can't see the problem." (This is so true in public education and politics!)

T. S. Eliot stated, "Humankind cannot bear very much reality."

Leon Battista Alberti stated, "Men can do all things if they will."

Albert Einstein stated, "Great spirits have always found violent opposition from mediocrities." (This one from Einstein encompasses my whole public teaching career!)

There are many outstanding and observed true sayings that Kubik listed in his book, so I will just share one more. Alfred North Whitehead stated, "It requires a very unusual mind to make an analysis of the obvious."

Cardiovascular Doctrine
Creates a Mess

Fitness is and has been clearly misunderstood in the US. That being said, the issue can be directly pinpointed to 1965 and Kenneth Cooper's cardiovascular doctrine.

A shift in fitness occurred in the United States compared to the East after World War II. Cooper (1968 p25) stated, "If it's muscles or a body beautiful, you'll get it from weightlifting but not much more…If it's the overall health of your body you're interested in, isometrics won't do it for you, neither will isotonics or anaerobics. Aerobic exercises are the only ones that will." Dr. Kenneth Cooper, father of the aerobics craze, had stressed in his book, *Antioxidant Revolution*, that excessive amounts of strenuous endurance exercise may even make one more likely to contract heart disease and cancer because this short of activity causes a great increase in potentially harmful free radicals in the body. Authorities generally qualify their support for this fallacy by stipulating that the exercise has to be moderate,

> but this does not let them off the hook. This is the most difficult part of the process. It requires great skill to determine 'moderation' for each individual. Even then, moderate running in polluted cities often leads to respiratory problems, and moderate unskilled training in the gym often produces niggling injuries. The immune response in serious runners is seriously lowered while aerobic instructors frequently have limb or back pain or injury. (Siff 2003)

This is where the United States chose the wrong path, and this has led to many myths, fallacies, fads, and widespread misrepresentation of what fitness actually is. This has also led to many corrupt practices with insurance companies, hospitals, and government agencies walking hand in hand in complete misrepresentation of health, wellness, and nutritional guidelines.

"It was inevitable that the accompanying high profile marketing and media campaigns, extensively underwritten by the medical profession, would make the pursuit of strength-oriented sports considerably less attractive in the public eye" (Siff 2003). All these led to big money and self-promotion and ridiculous misstatements that became facts based on myths for over sixty years and counting: "squatting is bad for your knees," "lifting makes you slow," "girls can do push-ups on their knees," "walk ten thousand steps for health and fitness," "sport-specific lifting," "FitGram testing for physical education," "circuit training," "Tae Bo," "gazelle," "heart rate monitors," "moderate cardiovascular activity," "improving VO2 max will improve running performance," "functional training," "core training," or just buy a $1,500 Peloton bike to be fit (ha ha). I think you get the idea!

Proprietary programming can be described as taking a body of knowledge and packaging it for money. Many times, this leads to political corruption and questionable ethics and morality issues. These programs often create issues with how people perceive the information as well. The echo chambers that come out of these programs portray themselves as experts and become self-proclaimed champions of their cause, but unfortunately, they see the solution, but they do not see the problem. Self-promoting philosophies and money become the end result at the expense of factual knowledge and high-quality education. If junk science is taught to the future teachers, coaches, etc., then, obviously, the idea of education becomes a huge problem because the actual information learned is incorrect. This obviously becomes a detrimental problem, and that is exactly what has occurred in fitness, education, and coaching.

"We live in an era where supposed leaders appear to engage in a perpetual quest for the magic bullet of success." This is not more evident than in public education, fitness, and sport. Every year, in teaching, we have an in-service with the next magic curriculum, and the administrators in charge just keep drinking the Kool-Aid, and the kids suffer for the experts' ignorance and lack of leadership. "Society cannot handle too much common sense." Great teachers/coaches, both in fitness and education, are successful and find unmatching success without the assistance of externally imposed methods of instruction. Great teachers/coaches do not need special textbooks, curriculum, or secret information to achieve success.

The average fitness devotee wants quick fixes that require little additional work or single-minded concentration. The mind will involve itself in training to a greater extent if you simply allow the exercise to entice or seduce the mind into committing itself more sincerely to the action. How strongly does the mind become involved in any gym exercise if you use light, unchallenging movements, loads, reps, sets, and workouts (i.e., cardiovascular doctrine)? Under those conditions, the mind can go on holiday, keep almost entirely out of the training process, and even allow you to read, talk, or watch TV while you are exercising. Let's move to the opposite scenario. Use heavyweights, high-intensity training methods, heavy, super-slow—near maximal loads—reps to failure, novel training variations, concentration curls, minimal rest intervals, and other very demanding or challenging training strategies. Under these conditions…Can you let the mind relax, take a hike elsewhere, or watch TV and complete the exercise effectively? Not a chance! (Siff 2003)

When comparing free weight exercise to machines, it is very clear that free weights are vastly superior regardless of opinion but rather this is absolutely true scientifically and practically. Free weight exercise helps to increase bone density, tendon and ligament strength, and typically is multi-joint rather than single joint. Free weights work many muscles at one time (e.g., primary movers, stabilizers, etc.). Free weights deal with real-world movement. I watched my mother playing on the floor with my newborn son in his early years, and I loved watching her getting up off the floor holding the child using a single leg squat to get up at sixty-eight years old. I have seen many eighteen-year-olds who would struggle doing that. It is not a leap to suggest that the cardiovascular doctrine easily led the United States into the obesity epidemic and big pharmaceutical-driven messaging we see today. Free weights can be extremely aerobic yet with all the other benefits. "Eight benefits from the back squat by itself are improved bone density, increased muscle mass, increase in strength and stamina and performance in other areas of exercise, greater mobility, enhanced cardiovascular health, better mental health and enhanced moods due to release of endorphins during execution of the exercise, reduced risk of injury due to increased strength, and improved stability in joints" (Hudson 2022).

Free weights are tremendous for burning calories, losing weight, and most importantly, for gaining lean mass. This statement alone demonstrates that the whole BMI craze led by the medical community and federal government that totally ignores the lean muscle calculation speaks for itself. It is completely irrelevant unless directly relating the calculation to very obese individuals. It's amazing how the public schools, for many years, had to send BMI reports annually to parents, demonstrating what their children's BMI currently is. Most parents had little clue what was the truth from fact. I stated this fact to the department head at my school as well as my colleagues, and all just shrugged their shoulders and acknowledged that the state mandates it, so we should just go along. This is what goes on in public schools every day, and yet every adult follows that status quo line that they are doing what is best for the kids. The very professionals with degrees keep selling the snake oil fully aware that the information is the furthest thing from being correct or intelligent.

I also would argue that it could easily fail the Sandusky law in Pennsylvania, but again, the so-called educational gurus keep on picking and choosing what to follow under the guise of intelligence with a degree in the best interest of the children. My son was a high-level hockey player in middle school at the time, and I received his BMI, and it stated that he was one percent from being obese. Ironically, he was five feet five and 145 pounds at the time. He parallel squatted 245 pounds and was literally complete muscle, but according to BMI, he was almost obese. Good thing I knew to throw the paper in the garbage. At least it gave me the opportunity to teach my son the many political agendas and misinformation that exists on a daily basis.

Julie Appleby wrote a news article in khn.org in 2022 specifically addressing this very point. Ironically, the above example I was fighting was all the way back in 2004. The high math skills I possess say to me that this is eighteen years later, and the snake oil never went away, which says it all. The title of Julie's article is "BMI: The Mismeasurement of Weight and the Mistreatment of Obesity."

> People who seek medical treatment for obesity or an eating disorder do so with the hope their health plan will pay for part of it. But whether it's covered often comes down to a measure invented almost two hundred years ago by a Belgian mathematician as part of his quest to use statistics to define the 'average man.' (Appleby 2022)

Here we go with math and statistics again, and that snake oil was two hundred years ago, and the follow-the-science mantra is alive and well!

> That work done in the 1830s appealed to life insurance companies that created "ideal" weight tables after the turn of the century. By the 1970s and 1980s, the measurement, now dubbed body mass index, was adopted to screen for and track obesity. But critics—and they are widespread these days—say it was never meant as a health diagnostic tool. "BMI does not come from science or medicine," said Dr. Fatima Stanford, an obesity medicine specialist and the equity director of the endocrine division at Massachusetts General Hospital. (Appleby 2022)

> She and other experts said BMI can be useful in tracking population-wide weight trends, but it falls short by failing to account for differences among ethnic groups, and it can target some people, including athletes, as overweight or obese because it does not distinguish between muscle mass and fat.

Exactly my example above and exactly what I argued in 2004 and yet here we are in 2022, and education itself taught millions of children and parents completely wrong, and it was supported by medical professionals, state and federal government, school boards, and public schools. All these entities love to promote themselves in proprietary programming of fitness centers with expensive machines (especially in physical education programs) and pass this off as great education. My expert opinion says this is corrupt and wrong, but in systems thinking, everyone's opinion is equal, which hopefully this book shows you that things have to change, and fitness is one of the many places the snake oil needs to be exposed. I understood all of these because of my training time with Coach Stucky. Transformational knowledge indeed!

> Still, BMI has become a standard tool to determine who is most at risk of the health consequences of excess weight—and who qualifies for often-expensive treatments. Despite the debate surrounding BMI, the consensus is that people who are overweight or obese are at greater risk for a host of health problems, including diabetes, liver problems, osteoarthritis, high blood pressure, sleep apnea, and cardiovascular problems. (Appleby 2022)

Not sure how there is a debate on this topic? The whole echo chamber for BMI is astonishingly clear, and as you will see in a later chapter in this book, training the way I learned from Coach Stucky answers all the above issues with no medicine, and a longtime friend is the example I used to make it clear.

Let's get back to the corruption of big *pharma* and the insurance companies.

> The BMI measure is commonly included in the prescribing directions for weight loss drugs. Some of the newest and most effective drugs, such as Wegovy, limit use to patients who have a BMI of thirty or higher (i.e., the obesity threshold) or a lower level of twenty-seven if the patient has at least one weight-related medical condition, such as diabetes. Doctors can prescribe the medications to patients who don't meet those label requirements, but insurers might not cover any of the cost. While most insurers, including Medicare, cover some forms of bariatric surgery for weight loss, they might require a patient to have a BMI of at least thirty-five, along with

other health conditions, such as high blood pressure or diabetes, to qualify. (Appleby 2022)

With medications, it can be even trickier. Medicare, for example, does not cover most prescription weight loss drugs, although it will cover behavioral health treatments and obesity screening. Coverage for weight loss medications varies among private health plans. "It's frustrating because everything we do in obesity medicine is based on these cutoffs," said Stanford.

Critics say that BMI can err on both ends of the scale, mistakenly labeling some larger people as unhealthy and people who weigh less as healthy, even if they need medical treatment. For eating disorders, insurers often use BMI to make coverage decisions and can limit treatment to only those who rank as underweight, missing others who need help," said Serena Nangia, communications director for Project HEAL, a nonprofit that helps patients get treatment, whether they are uninsured or have been denied care through their health plan. "Because there's such a focus on BMI numbers, we are missing people who could have gotten help earlier, even if they are at a medium BMI," Nangia said. "If they are not underweight, they are not taken seriously, and their behaviors are overlooked."

Stanford said she, too, often battles insurance companies over who qualifies for overweight treatment based on BMI definitions, especially some of the newer pricier weight loss medications, which can cost more than $1,500 a month. [As you will discover throughout this book, $1,500 medications, $1,500–$2,500 Peloton bikes, walking ten thousand steps, etc.

does not solve the obesity epidemic. Lifting free weights as all clients in Force 46 Strength and Conditioning do along with how we add nutrition later in the program is our answer to all the echo chamber debates, proprietary programs, self-promotion, educational and governmental corruption, ignorance, and trying to solve problems with medicine. Something Coach Stucky knew many years ago!]

"The health of a person with a twenty-nine BMI might be worse than one with a fifty if that person with the twenty-nine has high cholesterol, diabetes, sleep apnea, or a laundry list of things," said Stanford, "while the person with a fifty just has high blood pressure. Which one is sicker? I would say the person with more metabolic disease."

Additionally, BMI can overestimate obesity for tall people and underestimate it for short ones, experts say. And it does not account for gender and ethnic differences.

Experts generally agree that BMI should not be the only measure to assess patients' health and weight. "It does have limitations," said David Creel, a psychologist and registered dietitian at Cleveland Clinic's Bariatric and Metabolic Institute. "It doesn't tell us anything about the difference between muscle and fat weight." Noting that many athletes might score in the overweight category or even land in the obesity range due to muscle bulk.

Instead of relying on BMI, physicians and patients should consider other factors in the weight equation. One is being aware of where weight is distributed. Studies have shown that health risks increase if a person carries excess weight in the midsection. "If someone has thick legs and most of their weight is in the lower body, it's not nearly as harmful as if they have it around their midsection, especially their organs," said Creel.

Stanford agrees, saying midsection weight "is a much better proxy for health than BMI itself," with the potential for developing conditions like fatty liver disease or diabetes "directly correlated with waist size."

New ways to define and diagnose obesity are in the works, including a panel of international experts convened by the prestigious Lancet Commission," said Stanford, a member of the group. "Any new criteria ultimately approved might not only help inform physicians and patients, but also affect insurance coverage and public health interventions.

Stanford has also studied a way to recalibrate BMI to reflect gender and ethnic differences. It incorporates various groups' risk factors for conditions such as diabetes, high blood pressure, and high cholesterol. Based on her research, she said, the BMI cutoff would trend lower for men as well as Hispanic and White women. It would shift to slightly higher cutoffs for Black women (Hispanic people can be of any race or combination of races). "We do not plan to eliminate the BMI, but we plan to devise other strategies to evaluate the health associated with weight status," said Stanford. (Appleby 2022)

This sums up another truly remarkable script that seems to occur at every corner of society (ills of society). For all the educational expertise and well-meaning of some, in the end, a panel of international experts will convene to discuss in a likely echo chamber or circle jerk, if you prefer, and the final quote is, "We do not plan to eliminate the BMI, but we plan to devise other strategies to evaluate the health associated with weight status" (Appleby 2022). This is status quo but well-meaning, and I understand this. Likely, many of the credentialed people are likely good people. But again, if people are educated and they clearly point out the issues with the concept of BMI, then why do we need to have an international meeting stating that they do not plan on eliminating the BMI but they plan to devise other strategies to evaluate the health associated with weight status? The real issue is muscle mass, and if people were actually educated with the background of strength and conditioning from experts like Coach Stucky, which I have taught for over thirty years, then many of the issues in this article would go away. Likely the red tape and corruption within big medicine, insurance companies, and dishonest theories like BMI might go away as well. Free weights lifted in our way do not discriminate by gender or body type or underlying conditions. In all cases to this point, I control my diabetes by lifting like this, I totally reversed my cholesterol curve as have some my clients and some in a short time have been able to get off high blood pressure medicine.

If we, as a society, want to really get at these health and fitness problems, then the experts like Coach Stucky with knowledge base of strength and conditioning and program design have to be finally recognized. This was a major goal of this book. Physical education programs in public schools then become of great importance and how they are structured. My wife and I have done this along with a grading system applied from the S-factors from Siff and Verkhoshansky (2003) as discussed in the physical education chapter in our book.

Lastly, to try to beat this point into the ground, free weight exercise improves flexibility and of great importance is tremendous for dynamic flexibility.

Machines, in the classic sense (not reverse hypers or back extensions etc.), typically work single joints. Machines typically are not weight bearing. Machines are not structural and accomplish the work for the lifter. Typically, machines do not work the stabilizing muscles. Stiff 2003 noted that it would typically take twelve to fifteen machines to attempt to equal the work in the back squat [or kettlebell snatch and likely all those machines would not be as effective]. The idea that machines are a great form of exercise is really the furthest thing from scientific fact just like the cardiovascular doctrine, BMI, and standardized testing does not correlate to any real truth. It is, in short, corruption, ignorance, and a lie.

[Research alone in this has been designed poorly and improperly interpreted but taken as fact. The following studies in Siff 2003, dismantle the cardiovascular doctrine, yet you would be hard-pressed to find any people who have been taught this information unless they were exposed to top strength and conditioning coaches.] It was found that VO_2 max in elite runners was virtually the same over a forty-year period, yet performances continually increased over the forty years. Scientists found that performance was not based on VO_2 max but rather increased performance comes from the muscular level. It is more important what the muscles do with the available O_2 rather than increasing the amount of O_2 taken in. (Siff 2003)

The cardiovascular doctrine gave birth to noncompetitive gym aerobics, long-distance jogging and cycling. Manufacturers of sporting goods created fashion wear and equipment. Exercise soon became a status symbol to many who previously would never have considered perspiring for the sake of appearance and well-being. In fact, some of the most thorough research to analyze the effect of exercise on cardiac health revealed that regular, vigorous exercise significantly reduced the risk of first heart attack, irrespective of the type of activity.

The author of the study, Dr. R. Paffenbarger of Stanford University, examined two different populations over many decades: Harvard graduates who exercised in their leisure time and San Francisco longshoremen (dockworkers) who exercised vigorously as part of their work. He discovered that the risk of fatal heart attack among longshoremen was reduced by 50 percent for a weekly energy expenditure of 9,500 kilocalories. The Harvard study revealed that men who climbed at least fifty steps each working day displayed a 20 percent lower risk of first heart attack. In general, those in this group expending more than 8,400 kilocalories of energy per week in leisure time activity had a 39 percent lower cardiac risk. The findings of the longshoremen study clearly demonstrate that the strenuous, sporadic resistance activity that characterizes dock work has a profoundly beneficial effect on the heart. (Siff 2003)

These studies demonstrate how the cardiovascular doctrine had a large echo chamber in the United States that ignored this kind of science and had the backing of the big hospitals and insurance companies. To this day, I still see the long slow distance coaches running kids mile after mile, which has little to no positive effect on the poor athletes' sports performance, and little has changed in many of the towns across the country.

I had firsthand knowledge of the next chapter in the cardiovascular doctrine with the new PE. PE4life became the new mantra in school that followed the cardiovascular doctrine and engaged in epic proprietary programming and self-promotion. The big craze was to create huge fitness centers that often required grant money and kids working out on machines and walking with pedometers. Incorporating outdoor education as being great fitness along with team building became just as ridiculous as the long slow distance gurus for cardiac health. The brilliant new physical educators along with many others involved in this echo chamber tried to pass the target heart rate training to push their agenda. I'll go into more detail in the new PE chapter, however, in short, the idea that training over your maximum heart rate is not safe is truly nonsense and driven by a large group of people who should not be teaching fitness or training kids specifically.

Many of the people I saw were individuals who were not even fit themselves, yet they all were shouting at the top of the mountain with junk science that they were helping in teaching kids to be fit. As you read this book, you will clearly see that their echo chamber does not even know the science of what makes up fitness; and clearly, the corruption followed the script of the cardiovascular doctrine. I especially took issue with this because I was the Pennsylvania state director for the NSCA at the time and completed all my graduate-level work in exercise and sport studies along with having been trained by the best college strength coach at the University of Arkansas (John Stucky). I was appalled at the behavior of the new PE teachers' ignorance, and yet they all walked around with fake stature and no clue or care.

The target heart rate zone is about as beneficial as the body mass index (BMI). It is also as worthless as the cardiovascular doctrine. I can remember PE teachers and PE conferences stating that the PACER test was a great fitness test (which it is not), and that the kids should stop if they get over 185 on their watch. This arbitrary number also changed over the next couple of years but not sure what part of the cult made the decision for the next magic number for the PACER test!

Siff pointed out that in the lighthearted situation of heightened passionate encounter between two lovers, even at the fairly physically undemanding level of kissing, the heart rate of both parties can remain above 140 beats per minute for prolonged periods of time. The above formula would then imply, for a couple in their early twenties, that the activity involved is providing cardiovascular conditioning at the intermediate level of intensity.

Siff 2003 cites another contrary study to the cardiovascular doctrine and target heart rate issue that is very significant. It is the observation that the heart rate of motor and motorcycle racing drivers can remain at a level exceeding 180 beats per minute for the duration of races often lasting several hours and reach two hundred beats per minute for transient phases of extreme competitiveness. Yet the incidence of traumatic cardiac episodes during these events is extremely low. For drivers of forty years of age, the above equations suggest that they are operating at their maximal heart rate for much of the race and at more than 110 percent of their maximum for significant periods. At this point, no amount of scientific revelation is likely to make the public approach the quest for health and beauty more rationally. It takes time for the general consciousness and educational standard of any society to advance to a higher level. In the meantime, the purveyors of the modern equivalents of snake oil are likely to continue making fortunes from the gullible and the lazy. (Siff 2003)

It is currently the year 2022 and little has changed or the fitness industry has become worse, so I guess there is more to write!

> [In the sport performance area,] the widespread Western use of classical periodization along the lines originally pioneered by Matveyev may create the impression that it should be regarded as the preeminent and most appropriate method of organizing long-term training. However, even among Russian researchers and scientists, this approach to training has attracted some fierce criticism (Verkhoshansky 1997). In particular, it has roundly criticized texts which extol so-called periodization breakthroughs, stating that the material being offered as an exact science is setting back the progress of training organization to the era of the 1950s. Verkhoshansky makes the interesting observation that many Westerners seem to be oblivious of the fact that the general paradigm of periodization was based

heavily on the philosophies and methodologies of communism.

The cyclical nature of periodization was strongly influenced by the five-year plans and other cycles of productivity in the Soviet system while the precise calculation of training quantities reflected attempts to minimize the unscientific factors of subjectivity and emotiveness. (Siff 2003)

It has been well documented that the Soviets dominated the United States in the Olympics in the sixties, seventies, and early eighties. Our experts observe the periodization and shock training concepts, and like usual, those two concepts get branded, promoted, and abused in the fitness industry even today. The first was Western Periodization. That became the training model of prominence up to at least 1997 and many still follow today. Ironically, information is always taken and then rebranded and packaged, in this case, we then get Western periodization so as to be different from the original Russian periodization concept. The second major insight I discovered was that our scientists found the Russians performing "shock" training typically done in the weight room (examples often done with the weightlifting exercises and kettlebells). Our ingenious scientists then came back to the United States and miraculously created the Russian shock training but making it to be performed with body weight. This packaging becomes termed plyometrics.

Siff clearly documented understanding plyometrics and how the West clearly exploited this training concept developed by Yuri Verkhoshansky.

Other than periodization, no other Russian sporting secret has captured the attention of Western coaches and athletes as powerfully as so-called plyometrics. This training method is commonly regarded as being most synonymous with depth jumps and medicine ball throws with virtually every book in the English language not discussing the difference between classical plyometrics and more conventional jumps. It is almost never mentioned that plyometrics may not even be necessary for certain athletes at certain stages of training or that it may be one of the less appropriate activities when offered inappropriately in the training of any athlete. However, even supporters of plyometrics may not be correct in fairly randomly and routinely introducing it into the training of every athlete, even if they follow some form of periodized exercise prescription. Even Western research is corroborating the finding that plyometrics appear to be most effective when combined in some concurrent or sequential way with other resistance training and not merely as a substitute for resistance training to produce greater explosive power. The actions of plyometrics occur very commonly during running, sprinting, hurdling, jumping, and numerous other sporting activities so that athletes regularly taking part in these activities may well be performing quite sufficient plyometric training. (Siff 2003)

The confusing realm of popular plyometrics as taught in the context of Western sport may conveniently be analyzed by reviewing the following two well-known textbooks on this subject in the light of their original Russian work that refined this training method in the 1960s: *Jumping into Plyometrics* by D. A. Chu, published in 1992 by Leisure Press, Champaign, Illinois, and *Plyometrics: Explosive Power Training* by J. C. Radcliffe and R. C. Farentinos, published in

1985 by Human Kinetics Publ. Inc., Champaign, Illinois. (Siff 2003)

These readable, well presented little volumes present an interesting array of jumping and rebound activities, many of which do not constitute true plyometric training as conceived by Russian scientists some thirty years ago. Such exercises are supplementary or preparatory movements that lead up to or accompany plyometric training, but they frequently are not true plyometrics drills as envisioned by their Russian pioneer. (Siff 2003)

Plyometrics is the Westernized term applied to what Russians call the "shock method." This is a technique characterized by impulsive action with a minimal duration between the end of the eccentric braking phase and the initiation of the concentric acceleration phase. The preface of Chu's book expresses his intention to dispel the myths and dispel the misinformation about plyometrics, and its cover announces that the book is the most complete book ever written on plyometrics, and that no one is more qualified to write about this form of explosive power training than Donald Chu despite the fact that Verkhoshansky is the unrivaled international pioneer in this field. (Siff 2003)

As Verkhoshansky is an unrivaled pioneer in training research and plyometrics, John Stucky is the unrivaled pioneer in strength and conditioning and program prescription.

No distinction is made between maximal and submaximal plyometrics (and how they are produced) nor is the concurrent and sequential prescription of plyometric and other forms of training discussed in any depth. For example, both books advocate sessions with over one hundred repetitions of plyometric movements, sometimes combined with resistance training. This volume of maximal plyometrics (unlike submaximal plyometrics) is neither feasible nor safe for any athlete. Maximal plyometrics, like maximal weightlifting, involves single all-out repetitions separated by a few minutes of rest. It is extremely demanding on the central nervous system and imposes great mechanical strain on the tendons in particular. (Siff 2003)

This begins the echo chamber of sport coaches who are not strength coaches and shout in a loud voice to their team that if you do depth jumps, then you will be more explosive and jump higher. Often, they do this with middle school and unprepared high school players who have many strength and flexibility deficiencies and yet hold strength and core sessions for untrained athletes in these training modes with absolutely no true concept other than they heard or read from books like Donald Chu that plyometrics are the next great thing. Of course, this then trickles down to the elementary flag football or swimming coach who starts implementing plyometrics at even earlier ages because now everyone wants to get an NIL deal, and the train wreck continues with no end in sight.

Many of the so-called great strength and conditioning coaches today will promote what they do with their athletes, and typically, it's the national champion or blue-blooded teams. The higher-level coaches will promote/present the many training drills such as specific lifts, speed drills, and practice schemes with their high profiled athletes, which entices the novice high school and below coaches who typically did not even play the sport they are coaching at a very high level bring the drills back to the kids and use the snake oil words of this is how you get better. These admirers fail to realize that the kids these division I coaches are already coaching really talented athletes who already run sub 4.5 forties, so the application of what the national champions are doing is not what beginning athletes should be doing. This is just a simple observation I have seen for more than thirty years, but it's just one of many problems going on in training and fitness today.

> Western plyometric supporters and self-proclaimed experts also strongly criticize the recommendation that athletes should be able to squat 1.5–2 times body mass to use certain plyometric drills since they consider that this criterion is not based on research evidence and does not apply to all plyometric exercises. This recommendation is a safety measure based on force plate analysis of maximal plyometrics in the form of depth jumps where the ground reaction force on the lower extremity can easily exceed six times body weight. (Siff 2003)

Do not get confused because actual weight room ability is important with submaximal plyometrics as well and how they are segmented and total volume of repetitions, etc. Athletes who cannot properly deep squat their body weight and demonstrate they have good dynamic flexibility and overall motor control really have no business doing even submaximal plyometrics unless you are talking about basic elementary deceleration drills or skipping, galloping, etc.

> Certainly, the so-called plyometric drills in these books are known to enhance performance, but it is not predominantly due to plyometric action but more to the increased loading of eccentric contraction, the conditioning of connective tissue, the improvement of voluntary starting strength from the quasi-isometric state, and enhancement of acceleration strength by increasing the velocity of projectiles such as medicine balls. (Siff 2003)

These distinctions should be part of any physical education program and strength and conditioning program, and yet I have come across very few who even have a clue on this discussion. They just hear plyometrics are good and off they go training the next great six-year-old. "With regard to plyometrics, it is better to leave a power tool alone if you have no clue how to use it" (Tsatsouline 2001).

If you add Kenneth Cooper's cardiovascular doctrine along with the above examples, you should be able to have the light bulb come on in your head! This is where I appreciate Coach Stucky even more! Coach Stucky was a pioneer in strength and conditioning at the division I level in the 1970s. My story of improvement actually paralleled his in that my abilities dramatically improved because of his knowledge of what lifting can do for athletes. To this day, I have not met any strength coach who could compare to the man Coach Stucky was, and I think about him every day! It is the knowledge I gained from training under Coach Stucky that allowed me to be able to develop program design for fitness, athletic ability, mental health and wellness and to develop the best physical education program for public schools.

Western periodization is another Western promoted take on Russian expertise. Verkhoshanky (1997) pointed out that the typical mechanical division of annual training into periods and mesocycles has been based on the short-term experience of preparation of athletes during the early stage of formulating the Soviet system of training (of the 1950s) and mainly on the example of three sports (swimming, weightlifting, and track-and-field). Therefore, the annual training into periods and mesocycles cannot be universally applied in its basic form. It is emphasized that any system of training should be based not so much on logic and empirical experience but much more on physiology (Siff 2003).

With all the education I have had, I can tell you that my knowledge on program design truly came from training (physically performing) under Coach Stucky at the University of Arkansas as the biggest influence. Working under Joe Kenn at Boise State University was of great benefit, as well as reading the Russian manuals (which was never part of any curriculum), and reading the strongman books of Hackenschmidt and Kubik really helped drive my philosophy. There is no true book on program design. Those few who strive to get out of the box with proven experience and are fortunate to have been able to learn from actual pioneers in training are the individuals who people need to learn from to get rid of proprietary programming and politically fake science. This will allow for more clarity and the benefit for our children's future. This was a big goal of mine with the writing of this book.

Many experts have been promoted and supported in the proprietary programming mode. We have many who sided with Western periodization. We have had many who sided with Undulating periodization; we currently have the conjugate method disciples. We have the Cooper Institute disciples (which I would give no credence to). We had the HIT method (one set to failure echo chamber… LOL). They all have shown benefits and success stories, but in the end, following all these echo chambers becomes the proverbial "circle jerk," and more progressive ideas and approaches get ignored or stifled. Simply put, this is exactly what public education has become. Frivolous information tied up with politics and ignorance that becomes nothing but a "circle jerk!"

Force 46 physical education is our way to take aim at this "circle jerk" (e.g., coaching and physical education) and create great physical education and strength and conditioning possibilities for all schools and all people in all fifty states. However, if this book inspires only one teacher or school or regular person wanting to move through life with ease, then we can be happy because whoever begins to understand what we are saying will allow all types of people to improve and be happy, and this would be a great thing. This example in training also occurs in physical education.

AAHPERD (the American Alliance for Health, Physical Education, Recreation, and Dance) PE4life, which now has moved to SHAPE America, all preach the same doctrine, all preach the same words. The names change, but because there is corruption and politics in it, the message always fails, and the rehash of the same trash will find a new name and repeat its sins. The physical education program my wife and I developed follows none of these groups, and we developed the ideas with over fifty-five years of success based on much research and experience with the goal of what is best for kids and getting rid of the fluff and junk agendas.

To piggyback off this same premise, I found an article written by Alex Hughes. The title of the article is "HIIT versus Weight Training: Which Will Make You Fitter? A Physiotherapist Explains the Difference." I recall back in the 1990s and early 2000s, the HIT method was being promoted specifically by Ken Mannie from Michigan State University. Penn State University and the Washington Redskins strength gurus were also prevalent in this theory of one set to failure. The people I was around with and I never gave any credence to this echo chamber, but as with all things identified throughout this book, all kinds of theories / echo chambers and self-promoters gather a following and take a place at the mountaintop to push their belief. Ironically, when you read all the science cited in the book, it becomes very clear that one set to failure is no real way to train at all and could never address all the facets that real strength and conditioning needs to offer on a weekly basis.

As science disproved the original HIT method, years later, we now have a new model called HIIT training. Conveniently, an extra I has been added to the old HIT method. The added I is interval training. Hughes stated that "while both are legitimate options in the gym, they are very different in their results and styles. HIIT is an exercise routine that works in short intervals of high-intensity movement. The actual exercise varies but can often include bodyweight exercise, sprinting, biking, and other similar moves. Weight training, on the other hand, is the use of weights to improve your strength." Here we go again. Weight training is for strength? "What strength are we talking about?" should be one of the first questions that comes to mind.

"If you are looking to build absolute strength, then weight/resistance training would be the best option," said Dr. Luke Connolly, a lecturer in physiotherapy at Plymouth University. "However, if you're a complete beginner when it comes to exercise, you could find HIIT or weight training could feel like a very serious jump." The high-intensity nature of interval training can be somewhat uncomfortable to begin with, so it is advised for absolute beginners that they become accustomed to MICT (i.e., medium-intensity continuous training) first before trying HIIT (Hughes 2022). LOL! The new jargon coming out of the latest brilliance of fitness seems to have a lot of acronyms. Some questions I have about this new knowledge is, What is high intensity? The last time I checked, lifting maximal weights was very intense. The last time I checked, doing kettlebell Russian ladders was very intense. The last time I checked, doing a squat clean at a moderately heavy load was intense. The last time I checked, the movement speed of the lift can dictate how intense the activity is and that differing muscles will be taxed more depending on that speed.

The newfound high-intensity interval training appears to be more geared to the cardiovascular doctrine and even elements of CrossFit where appropriate rep ranges are ignored as well as rest intervals. To make matters worse, I am sure universities and certifications are creating testing questions on this nonsense, which clearly indicates that many individuals who are certified are actually not certified in any real knowledge of appropriate training. Again, if you want to focus on keeping your heart rate up, you can do that by running up and down your steps for one minute straight…not really sure how that constitutes training of any real benefit, but hey, be my guest.

Program design is of utmost importance (e.g., where you place exercises, what exercises to use, how many reps, and the ability to not overtrain weekly on a year-to-year basis). While many training schemes and types of lifts with different equipment will show benefits (especially in beginner level or novice individuals), lifelong training that covers all the bases is really what I am referring to. Social media and YouTube are completely filled daily with fitness influencers. And when most of the general public does not have the ability to recognize who is really good versus who is just wanting their fifteen minutes of fame or who is just plain wrong, then very strange belief systems from total inexperience become obstacles. The body-shaping crowd, cardiovascular doctrine crowd, powerlifting crowd, drug-induced crowd, nondrug crowd, gear crowd, raw crowd, weight loss crowd, and competition crowd (i.e., CrossFit games crowd) all claim snippets of how to train. As the science and experience in this book is presented, it should be a guide to knowing what is really good training and what is false advertisement. Coach Stucky was the best at this in his theories, beliefs, and design and that helped drive what we believe to be the best way to train and to design training for the human body in any individual's personal pursuit. We get shredded lifting like this; we get great sport performance lifting like this; we lose weight lifting like this; we get mental health benefits lifting like this; we get extremely strong in all realms of strength and flexibility lifting like this; we get great conditioning like this; and we get literally 100 percent adherence lifting like this.

The article addresses other concepts briefly that a real strength coach would understand is very inexperienced in the training realm and likely has never been exposed to the likes of a John Stucky. "Medium-intensity continuous training (e.g., jogging, cycling or pickup sports like tennis, squash or basketball) can be a good gateway for someone who isn't quite ready for the more demanding exercises of HIIT or weight training. After that, it is a question of whether your goals are more aligned with strength or cardiorespiratory fitness" (Hughes 2022). This completely is opposite of what we do at Force 46. We have a nine-week general prep done in the weight room designed to learn how to perform lifts in a sequence that can take any person (even from a level of zero) and focus on preparing the body to actually train all the while the person is actually training. To truly lift weights, one must continuously learn and perfect the form. The simplistic idea that once you start performing some lifts really well makes you an expert in this kind of training is not true. If you lift like this, you will be perfecting form and be mentally cognizant in every training session thirty years later. It never gets old, and you will always be challenged, and you can do it your entire life. I have trained an individual (Ben Amsler) who graduated as commander of the corp (highest ranking cadet) at West Point (as you will see later in the book), and we trained 90 percent of his so-called cardio ability in the weight room. Again, program design, teaching philosophy/ability, and understanding actual science from junk science will prevent you from joining an echo chamber that lives in a circle jerk.

The article's final statement is "the best exercise will come down to whether you're training strength or cardiovascular wellness." Coach Stucky and I would say why in the world are we not training both along with all the other aspects of fitness instead of just focusing on a fingernail's worth of fitness and claiming it is the end of all training program based on knowing the solution but in reality, not ever knowing or seeing the problem.

This then lead to a final article I read that is written very well, however, will lead to a different echo chamber in strength and conditioning, which will then trickle down to K-12 schools and will likely be skewed by differing perceptions and create new magic bullets and theories that likely will go very awry. The article was written by Lachlan James. The article is "Strength Testing and Training: Understanding Which Strength Quality to Focus on."

> Over the last twenty years, there has been an exponential increase in availability of strength testing options. So when it comes to assessing the different classifications of strength, how should coaches see the wood through the trees? Lachlan James and a number of other authors recently published an update to their classic paper, "Strength Classification and Diagnosis: Not All Strength Is Created Equal." So we asked Lachlan six questions to pull out the key points.

> Question 1: Are there any strength testing or training methods that you feel have become commonplace but are overhyped for whatever reason?

Lachlan answered that testing methods to a given situation should be objectively defined through a thorough needs analysis. This process will tell you what tests and metrics to focus on and, therefore, what training interventions are needed. He stated that often researchers and, consequently, practitioners miss this step. The process the authors promote is to look at strength qualities then competition performance indicators then competition outcomes. A needs analysis is always a good idea, but again, while it all sounds well and good, it's the knowledge and program structure on a daily basis that really yields the results both short term and long term, which you will see as we progress through this knowledge promotion. Also, the idea of spirit and skill has a huge impact on actual performance, so simply identifying strength qualities in an academic manner really follows the sport specificity echo chambers, which many follow as religiously as the cardiovascular doctrine echo chamber. The real issue I have observed for over thirty years of training from the division I level down is how the idea of specificity and sports has created many echo chambers still attempting to address concepts great strength coaches already knew and had been practicing. It is my opinion that Coach Stucky was the best at this, and it is not as complicated as many practitioners and academic physiologists make it out to be. I address throughout this book how periodization, plyometrics, sport specificity, and specialization have been misinterpreted and misused; and nothing has really changed over the last thirty years and counting, yet the next magic paradigm is presented as new, and in reality, it is the same rehash of old trash (i.e. scientific analysis and sport specificity to answer success). The article goes on to say, "This process will tell you what tests and metrics to focus on and, therefore, what training interventions are needed. Liaising with the sport scientist to establish the key performance indicators of your sport is an important first step. Those indicators themselves must be empirically linked to competition outcome (e.g. wins vs. losses, ladder position) (James 2022). [I believe and I have known for years that testing really comes down to absolute strength, speed-strength, explosive strength and strength endurance. Testing should not be complex and it is a very small part to a much bigger picture of what a true strength coach does. A perfect example of this is from an article written by Tom Murphy. The title of the article is "Barry Foster a Key Cog in Hatfield's Flexbone Offense"].

Foster's work ethic and dedication to the game made him life-long admirers during his three-year stint with the Razorbacks. "The thing I remember about Barry was he was a football player's player," Hatfield said. "He would come out, he'd work hard and he'd do everything you say. Then, when the day was over, he'd go back in with John Stucky our strength coach. John would load some weights up on a little sled and he would have Barry pull those things after practice when he was dead tired. "He just faithfully and religiously did that. I think it gave him not just confidence, but it gave him the power and the strength. In our offense, the key revolves around the fullback. You've got to have a good, strong person who is gonna get hit every time, even if he doesn't have the ball. So it takes a tough constitution to do that and Barry had it." Said Hatfield, "If you could draw up a mold, he would be one for playing that position. He was strong, he was tough, he had speed, he had great hands." Foster, a 5'10, 223-pounder at the height of his pro career, said the dive back in the Flexbone suited him magnificently. "It was perfect for my skill set," he said. "I wasn't an overly fast guy, even though I could play tailback, which I did for the University of Arkansas, I was much more comfortable between the guard and the tackle. "I was a shorter, squatty guy, big strong shoulders. So I really excelled at going with the quick dive play off the tackle and stuff like that." (Murphy 2022)

As you can see from the above example, it is less about the sport and more about the players when it comes to a great strength and conditioning program and that is something Coach Stucky understood back in the 1970s. Barry Foster pulling a sled after practice is classic Coach Stucky, and hopefully this helps you understand that great training is far more than sport specificity and scientific testing and metrics when it comes to great performance.

My good friend Todd Burkey spoke about needs analysis twenty-four years ago, so this is not something that should be new to any strength coach. However, this article makes it sound like it is new. Siff stated that all human movement can be simply broken down into four main types of strength—absolute strength, speed strength, explosive strength, and strength endurance (Siff 2003). Great strength programs address this even if a specific quality is more inherent than another. Also, the understanding of direct and indirect abilities, which I cite in the "Physical Education" chapter, is very important in the argument over how important specificity becomes. I have found that it is even more important to identify the needs analysis for the individual player more so than the sport that they are playing. We have to also take into account how this affects the multisport athlete. We then need to also take into serious consideration the idea of injury prevention, which should be the primary goal of a strength and conditioning program.

What I take from this particular article is that the researchers created a paradigm for analyzing the two most important strength qualities in a given sport, giving the most important strength quality as the primary training goal and then a secondary training goal of the next most specific strength quality. They created a simple chart outlining the identified strength quality and then listed the primary training and then secondary training. This is an idea that I would never follow. Here are some reasons why: In the sport of volleyball, there is a lot of reactive ability and explosive ability. According to the article, the primary training, for reactive strength, would be plyometric (fast SSC) and the secondary training would be plyometric (slow SSC) and heavy strength training. Volleyball by nature is very plyometric, and a strength coach has to be aware that trying to train plyometrics in the weight room will likely lead to overtraining because they are already doing that in practice. Second to this point, you may have a volleyball player who shows promise and has good explosive strength but is very weak in the absolute strength realm along with possibly needing strength endurance in the lower back and shoulders. In this example then, plyometric would not be the primary training emphasis, which is why I rarely base a training program with a paradigm based on the requisite strength qualities of a given sport. This really can be said for all sports. I also think that testing is currently becoming more complex than it needs to be and way too many variables become a problem, but that is the current trend. Lastly, psychological factors and the skill of the athlete really dictate the true success of a great program design.

> Question 2: What are the five strength and speed strength qualities that you feel should be tested and how?

The authors put all the multi-joint, lower body strength power tests in the mix and believed five unique, independent strength qualities (domains) appeared to emerge. The five strength qualities as defined by these authors are maximal isometric strength, explosive strength, fast dynamic strength, heavy dynamic strength, and reactive strength. In their view, the needs analysis process outlined above dictates the decision on which strength qualities to include in a testing battery.

The authors defined maximal isometric strength as the greatest amount of force applied to an immovable object regardless of the rate or ability to sustain the effort. "Practitioners can assess this via the isometric mid-thigh pull (IMTP) or isometric squat" (James 2022). Here we go with acronyms again. Explosive strength is defined by these authors as the slope of the initial portion of the force-time curve generated by the IMTP or isometric squat. They also stated in research settings that explosive strength is typically referred to as the rate of force development (RFD) or fast/rapid force production. Fast dynamic strength is defined by these authors as force expressed maximally against no or little external load over relatively long movement times (greater than three hundred ms). Common assessments are the countermovement jump (CMJ) or squat jump. Heavy dynamic strength is defined by these authors as force expressed against heavy loads, most often via a one or three RM primary lift like a squat or dead lift. "We can also assess heavy dynamic strength via the repetition velocity of a heavy but submaximal load (80–90 percent of 1RM) of a primary lift. It is important to note that heavy dynamic strength is distinct from maximal isometric strength, except in competitive weightlifters" (James 2022). Reactive strength is defined by these authors as the ability to tolerate and produce force in a fast (less than 250 ms) stretch shortening cycle action. The standard assessments are the drop jump or rebound jump with the cue to minimize contact time and maximize jump height. This, of course, is plyometrics, and I already outlined and described in detail, citing the work of Siff and Verkhoshansky as well as how this concept has been totally misrepresented in the West, so nothing new here.

> Question 3: When testing with equipment like force plates, we can collect countless metrics. However, what metrics within these tests should we focus on?

> Maximal isometric strength is an easy one. The metric of interest is peak force, which may or may not be scaled to body mass depending on the context. Explosive strength is quantified by the force, impulse or rate of force development (if reliable) at 150 ms or less in the IMTP or isometric squat. Durations greater than this threshold produce strength outputs that are too similar to maximal isometric strength to be considered a unique strength quality. (James 2022)

The authors' rule of thumb was to select the earliest time point that was reliable, which in their experience seemed to be force at one hundred ms.

> It is well documented that the CMJ assessment of fast dynamic strength can produce dozens of metrics. Data reduction procedures can

reduce them to one primary and one secondary domain. The primary domain includes measures such as jump height or peak velocity while the secondary domain seems to be represented by a timing metric such as time to take-off. Heavy dynamic strength is well known to practitioners via rep max (RM) and velocity testing. Eccentric and concentric-only variations of RM testing are available, but they don't tell you anything different from a conventional RM test. The reactive strength index derived from the drop jump or rebound jump is the key takeaway for reactive strength. Divide the jump height by the contact time and give feedback after each trial to make sure the contact time is less than 250 ms. (James 2022)

Question 4: For each of these qualities, are you able to give us any recommendations as to how to train each of them?

The authors stated that based on the principle of specificity, the training most similar to the testing task will have the greatest transfer. However, we have to consider other factors such as proper periodization, the athlete's existing capabilities, and the constraints of the training environment. The Russian weightlifting 1984 yearbook study that I will describe later should be a red flag for the sport specificity and plyometrics echo chamber along with Verkhoshansky's questioning of periodization in and of itself. Yet in the year 2022, we have researchers and PhD's writing articles scientifically rehashing the same ideas with big wording and really not ever getting outside the box. Specificity and plyometrics with young multi-sport athletes then becomes a huge problem when paradigms like this are created.

With this in mind, here is the author's general framework. The framework lists strength quality then primary training then secondary training. Maximal isometric strength quality would have a primary training of heavy strength training emphasizing a concentric start, end portion ROM, and a secondary training of maximal isometric tasks. The explosive strength quality would have weightlifting derivatives as the primary training and ballistic/plyometrics with minimal countermovement. The heavy maximal dynamic strength quality would have heavy strength training as the primary training and weightlifting derivatives as secondary training. The fast maximal dynamic strength quality would have plyometric (slow SSC) as the primary training and heavy strength training and weightlifting derivatives as the secondary training. Finally, the reactive strength quality would have the plyometric (fast SSC) as the primary training and plyometrics (slow SSC) and heavy strength training as the secondary training.

Hopefully, you are realizing now how the scientific echo chambers use educational big words and models to push great knowledge, and this is the furthest concept of great training knowledge packaged as a proprietary program or paradigm. This is the kind of information that will be in the colleges and testing for future strength and conditioning coaches along with the professional bureaucracy of sports that will keep fueling the ridiculous self-promotion and training fads using talented athletes to try to verify the framework concept. This actually is the furthest thing from the truth, and yet the same rehash of old trash keeps being published. The real issue about these kinds of models is how this information is perceived (or taken as gospel) by communities that are filled with mom and dad coaches or coaches who were not great at high school sports but loved to believe they were the greatest. This becomes a huge problem because often the public schools themselves are also part of the problem, and when you get multisport athletes being told to train in completely improper ways by three different coaches, then the kids truly suffer!

> Question 5: Is there space for very sport specific tests within a battery? How can we ensure that these tests are reliable and valid and that we understand what constitutes real change within them?

The authors quoted the following:

> There is definitely a space for them, depending on the situation. Such tests are often forms of jump tests, like a running vertical jump off one or two legs in sports where jumping is a key technical aspect of performance. However, it's important for practitioners to understand that they can't simply make up a test or metric! We must first establish that the new metric or test generates unique information that preexisting measures do not. Then as discussed in the first point of this article, we need to draw the association to performance in the sport, and that association should ideally be stronger than what already exists in other metrics. Then practitioners must confirm that the test or metric is reliable within and between individuals and is sensitive to change across time. Finally, they must be able to conduct the test and analysis within the training environment.

> Question 6: What are the biggest mistakes you see young practitioners make and what advice would you give them to help?

> If you are doing a test using instrumentation, choose just two variables from that test and make sure they each contain unique information (i.e., have a very low correlation). Do not get distracted by the instrumentation and not coaching, cueing, and providing feedback to the athlete. Familiarize yourself extremely well with all the equipment and the testing protocols. Pilot, pilot, pilot. This will leave you with extra attention during testing to focus on the athletes them-

selves. The ability to manage large groups, think on the fly, and quickly adjust training sessions based on situational constraints (e.g., limited time/equipment). Have a plan A, B, C, and D in your toolbox. How do you acquire the knowledge to have multiple plans? Shadow experienced coaches (this is exactly true), experienced practitioners, and applied sport scientists for as long as possible and see how they handle it. The more situations and challenges you get exposed to in a low-risk environment, the more prepared you will be once you're solo in the wild. (James 2022)

While this article is well written and using some of the same terminology that Siff and Verkhoshansky have cited from 1950 to 2003, the real issue is that it still follows much of the same echo chambers in training and fitness that have been long-standing and follows the periodization schemes that, partially true, ignore the idea and truth about how periodization was developed by Matveyev in the Soviet Union and that Verkhoshansky clearly criticized. The educated opinion utilizes the classic abuse and misrepresentation used in the West for promoting plyometrics as a primary tool that we have clearly described and cited in detail. The educated opinion or theory is that sport specificity is a major requirement in this paradigm, and again, you will see shortly how the Russian weight lifting 1984 yearbook described how specialization of tests was blown away by the kettlebell groups. The real issue I am getting at is I have seen these specific paradigms prescribed mainly by exercise physiologists because the thought continues to always be that you have to look at the sport. However, it is my experience and belief that you should look at the weaknesses your athlete has because any great athlete is always going to be working on absolute strength, speed strength, explosive strength, and strength endurance continuously; and literally, every sport requires ability in these realms. The issue of weaknesses is important because you can have a group of athletes that need all four types of strength to be trained but one group may specifically need to get more mass as well so that is a priority regardless if the sport requires speed strength and strength endurance. Another group in the sport may need strength–speed, absolute strength, etc. Program design then becomes less about the requisite skills of the sport but rather more about the needs of the athletes you have.

Also, the quote from Pavel Tsatsouline's book, with respect to the sport specific tests to the kettlebell groups, stated that the Russian scientists could not explain the spectacular all-around fitness gains from the standpoint of specificity but were too practical to be fazed by this mystery. "Understanding is a delaying tactic…," as one novelist put it. "Do you want to understand how to swim or do you want to jump in and start swimming?" "Only people who are afraid of the water want to understand." "Other people jump in and get wet." These statements, along with many others, are exactly what Coach Stucky understood, and it was easily felt in his daily workouts. Western periodization created the idea that you work different strength qualities in different blocks of time in the annual plan that I realized was missing the boat thirty years ago. If you leave strength qualities that you just spent time building, then you detrain those strength quality gains. Louie Simmons understood this very well too. Coach Stucky also was a prime example of Brooks Kubik's statement that lifting and lifting design is an art, and if someone tries to sell you a scientific book on training, then hit them hard and run like hell.

While the authors did make a correct claim to not get too complicated in the testing, the ideas presented likely will create a testing craze on metrics, and the tests for important strength qualities are not overly complicated. Coach Stucky already had a simple and relevant testing protocol at certain points of the year, and those testing protocols are every bit valid and reliable today as they were in 1992. The authors made a great point to include level of ability, and age needs to be a part of the needs analysis. That is true, however, the concept of spirit and training skill is not addressed significantly, and those two factors alone will lead to winning and performance improvement. This is why analytics and testing numbers become an echo chamber for the professional bureaucracy that has overtaken sports today. The wording and names seem to change, but really, it's quantitatively the same thing the great strength coaches did thirty to fifty years ago. Some just do it better than others. I believe Coach Stucky would say, "You guys go ahead and spend your time standing on force plates and testing because, on Saturday, you will regret your choice!"

Program Design and the Reality of Weight Loss, Fitness, and Pushing Numbers

The issue with weight loss is plastered all over the news on a daily basis, and social media has multiplied this craze and inundation with confusing misinformation for self-interest, money, and to get their fifteen minutes of fame. The 1980s had jogging while wearing headbands and spandex created from the cardiovascular doctrine. Clearly, that hasn't worked, yet any fool knows how to jog, so you still see people forty-two years later attempting to lose weight, jogging down the street. My wife and I sit on the porch and watch these individuals and feel sorry for them but, at the same time, laugh and then shake our heads. My wife ran track at Penn State University, and she was a cross-country runner by nature but knows this nonsense has to stop. You also get the added echo chamber from the nutrition side. Now all we have to do is click on Google, and we can have thousands of claimed eating habits that will allow us to lose weight, yet the vast majority still end up creating the yo-yo diet effect.

The yo-yo diet creates weight loss at first and then, within six months, the individuals can't figure out why they gained the weight back. To further complicate the issue in the vast majority of the weight loss seekers mind is that the Internet and phones all give us pictures of how to transform our body, and those looks somehow become the selling point. The new push to lifting weights is finally more on the correct side, however, the same self-promoting philosophies and infatuation with muscle size and making it a competition takes over, and the misleading and confusion starts all over again. Chasing big numbers in lifts and bodybuilding are fine for those wanting to compete in those venues, but the way the whole thing is presented in all the many forms of social media is now creating a very similar problem following the likes of the cardiovascular doctrine or step aerobics or Western periodization or plyometrics or the Peloton bike, etc.

I follow very simple rules that I have learned through much studying and personal experience to get rid of all the rhetoric, junk science, and self-promotion. The reality is you need to build total body muscle and dynamic flexibility and throw away the weight scale until you actually take the time to get physically prepared to train. A person should take the time to prepare their body to train the correct way and realize that it is a process, and when done correctly, you never put the weight back on. There are trainers making huge money, claiming huge weight loss in a short period of time especially in the entertainment industry, and that is fine, however, the entertainment industry is fake and does not live in reality, and most of us know this. They are the last people who should be the face of actual fitness and training.

We lift free weights only and promote a well-structured program design that eliminates overtraining and allows all the mental health benefits from great appropriate training. We do not claim to be fancy, as Coach Stucky used to say. I remember seeing an article in a magazine when Coach Stucky was interviewed at the time they won the national championship at the University of Tennessee. The reporter asked Coach Stucky about his training for the newly crowned champions. The reporter posed the question, looking for the next magic bullet and buzzwords to understand the great accomplishment the team had earned. Coach Stucky's response was exactly as I remembered, "We don't get fancy, we bench and squat." I still smile thinking about that to this day! I am one of the very fortunate ones who knows that Coach was more complex with his training programs, but he was every bit old school and humble, and that is as it should be!

When you program design correctly, then it becomes an all-in-one training process, and that is exactly why I know what I know today because I actually lived it. We do not promote a program for getting shredded, we do not promote a program for weight loss, we do not promote a program for sport performance, we do not promote clicking on another program designed for strength. If you lift like we do, our philosophical program does all of the above, and that is because the program's belief and design is the way it should be, and Coach Stucky was the creator.

I have trained so many success stories and go about it quietly just like Coach Stucky did, so I am only going to use one example for this book with respect to weight loss. When I decided to retire early from teaching to start my business for the pursuit of happiness/purpose and sharing my expertise, I contacted my longtime friend, Gary McCollough. He is a golf pro and a tremendous golf pro he is! Gary and I grew up together across the street from each other and have known each other since we were five years old. I hadn't seen Gary often over the last thirty years, but thankfully (on many levels), we have reunited.

Gary had been struggling with being very overweight, high blood pressure, aches and pains so bad that a chiropractor was a common monthly grab for help. I told him about my new business, and he joined in October of 2021. He told me just before starting that he was fully aware that he was going to die and felt like there was no help for him. I am writing this piece currently in September 2022. He has been lifting with me at 5:45 in the morning just under a year now.

In short, Gary was 215 lbs. and falling apart in every aspect of life. It was even hard for him to play eighteen holes of golf, and he was still a very good golfer, but he usually only played nine holes. I told him I believe in a nine-week general prep process in training to get the body ready to really train even though he will definitely see results and significant improvement even after three weeks. He definitely did see the improvement. The improvement not only was in his mobility and strength, but it was also his mental happiness as well.

About two months in, he said he felt so good but hadn't really lost weight. My response was to throw away the scale because weight doesn't matter right now. We need to build muscle and dynamic flexibility and work capacity, we can deal with weight soon. After about four to five months and he was feeling so much better. Gary's mind started to clear and then he was able to attack the nutrition aspect. He felt it was hard to change what and how you eat when you always feel horrible. Once he lifted long enough and his mind was so much clearer, the food was easy.

The enjoyment and learning of lifting made him want to fuel his body with good food instead of junk. Gary ended up increasing weight to 229 lbs. and had not had to see the chiropractor or doctor or anything and felt great. I knew he was like much of society, and they judge fitness by weight but it is about lean muscle, dynamic flexibility, and strength in the beginning and not weight simply put. Weight is irrelevant until you do the proper things on a consistent basis and train like me and Coach Stucky trained. I could visibly see the weight loss in him at the neck and shoulder first. I knew this was a good sign because he was losing weight in his upper body yet not on his magic scale. He faithfully lifted four days a week with me and loved every minute. He said he never was able to exercise more than a few weeks on any program and always quit. I smiled and said that is because the programs are junk and most of the so-called certified trainers have no idea. His only worry was the weight on the scale, so I started the nutrition piece with him. Gary currently has lost forty pounds, he is off high blood pressure medicine, never goes to a chiropractor, and has kept the weight off for exactly three more months during his crazy busy golf season, which is exactly what I told him in the beginning. When you train right and lose fat weight, you will never put the fat weight back on.

Gary's statement was, "If you decide that you just don't feel as good as you should and you are determined to change your habits, you can. Just get through the first nine weeks, and it's so much fun. You will thank yourself for sticking with it! What a great change physically, mentally, and spiritually it is! Training the force 46 way is the key to everything!" I can go into more detail, but things done right are rarely done in three weeks, we need to have a lifetime of improving and training the correct way to move through life. "When it is done correctly, it is the greatest feeling in the world, and I live it on a daily basis!"

New research from the University of Michigan suggests that people may want to invest in some weights and begin a strength training course. According to this research, weak muscles could be just as influential on your long-term health as smoking (Anderer 2022). This is something that I have been teaching and preaching about for over thirty years, however, as cited throughout this book, the cardiovascular doctrine disciples, along with all the corruption in the fitness industry, really ignored the value of free weights for years. Rather than repeat all the issues that have been raised, let's just focus on the positives from this research. The article stated the following:

> Not everyone ages at the same rate. Consider two adults, both sixty years old. While those two people may share the same chronological age, one may be far younger from a biological aging perspective. Aging is influenced by far more than days crossed off on the calendar. Genetic, environmental, and behavioral factors all play a major role as well. Poor lifestyle choices like avoiding exercise, unhealthy diet, and smoking are all believed to accelerate biological aging processes. Dealing with a serious illness can also age the body at an accelerated rate. (Anderer 2022)

"Now, for the first time ever, the team at the University of Michigan reports that muscle weakness marked by grip strength, a proxy for overall strength capacity, is connected with accelerated biological age. According to the findings, the weaker your grip strength, the older your biological age" (Anderer 2022). Obviously, by this point, the reader should realize that lifting free weights is the best thing for the human body, and again this is something that Coach Stucky understood even back in the 1960s. I was not born in the sixties but rather in 1971, so by 1992, after having the privilege of training under a true strength training pioneer and legend, I began to see all the ridiculous myths all the way to present time. This was a prime motivator for writing this book.

Force 46 Barrel

Recognizing what real science is versus junk science is very important. Otherwise, you will just be chasing your tail and reading headlines to support your incorrect opinion (e.g., cardiovascular doctrine disciple, etc.). Then taking that information and being able to apply that information to further improvement and increase the known science for the future is very important, but very few even get past the headlines and chasing one's tail. The ability to recognize what is good science versus junk science is also necessary, and most individuals fail at this, so the training protocols of belief systems spiral into the next wrong fad. Most just follow the status quo (mediocrities).

All the science cited so far—along with personal experience training under John Stucky and working the floor with Joe Kenn—and talking shop with other great strength coaches like Jerry Shreck from Bucknell, Todd Burkey (formerly from Youngstown State University), Jeremy Hoy (formerly from Finish First Sports, head Ohio state men's hockey), and longtime strength coach, Doug Smith (retired from Juniata College), really allowed me to develop the quest for better concepts in program design and prescription. Also, reading (and knowing who to read) information from greats like Brooks D. Kubik, Louie Simmons, Mel Siff, and Yurri Verkhoshansky is all relevant and needed to better training methods that haven't necessarily been studied in full in a laboratory setting. The creation of the force 46 barrel weights came from all this previous knowledge and what I believe is how program design should look like and how the human body should be trained.

The great diversity of human movements makes it necessary to evaluate the strength components of movements (submaximal strength, maximal strength, impulse strength, work and power), analyse the ability to produce strength (absolute strength, relative strength, and the moment of the force of muscular contraction about a joint), and to comparatively evaluate the strength components of movement (explosive strength, speed-strength movements, strength-endurance and others) which reflect the specificity of movements. Hence one is able to select appropriate methods for developing strength fitness.

Thus, muscular strength is a specific motor quality, and it is involved functionally under extremely diverse conditions in sport. Therefore, before discussing the methods of special strength preparation, the fundamental characteristics of producing muscular strength in sports movements must be examined.

Many studies have been devoted to the different regimes of muscular work. Based on the purpose of the work, they can be divided into two groups. One group is devoted to determining the conditions and regimes which increase the working effect of muscular strength, and the other to finding the regime which most effectively develops muscular strength. Unfortunately, many of these investigations have led to confusions and contradictions"

For example, some researchers maintain that the largest strength gains are made with dynamic (concentric) actions, others with isometric tension. Moreover, careful analysis of the experimental design reveals that similar contradictions are associated with invalid generalizations of results obtained in different laboratories, under unnatural conditions, on different muscle groups of subjects of different standards, using different loads and movement speeds. For instance, it was established that with maximal isometric tension of the biceps (elbow flexed at 90 degrees), subjects were able to develop a force 6.5–10.0 kg greater than the maximal weight that could be lifted concentrically.

However, this changes with a decrease in load and an increase in speed of movement. The electrical activity in the biceps muscle while lifting a weight of 50–80 percent of maximum is significantly greater than it is during the period when it is subsequently held statically, both in magnitude and the production of strength (Stepano and Burlakov, 1963; Monogarov and Laputin, 1966; Scheraev 1954, 1957; Rasch and Pierson, 1960; Yanchevsky and Steklove 1966).

Thus, there is an important difference in the characteristics of the muscular force displayed, depending upon the magnitude of the load and the speed of movement. It should be pointed out that the torque produced by the muscles increases approximately fourfold up to an angle of 90 degrees during elbow flexion. Therefore, for example, if you compare the force of a maximal isometric action developed at an angle of 90 degrees and the maximum weight which can be raised from an angle of 180°, then the force in the first case is greater. Consequently, if one is referring to the development of muscular strength, then to discuss superiority in the dynamic versus the isometric regime is scarcely appropriate because the biomechanical conditions for the production of strength are not comparable. If it is necessary to compare the training effect of a certain regime, then you must first establish which kind of strength is being measured. (Siff 2003)

Siff states:

Taking into consideration the diversity of sports activities, it is necessary to identify the specific character of the muscular tension, in particular, the different speeds with which tension is developed, its magnitude, duration, and number of repetitions as well as the state of the muscle preceding the working tension. To analyse all the diversity in sporting movements, muscular tension may be conveniently divided into at least eight types. This classification is central to the subsequent discussion of special strength training in sport. (Siff and Verkhoshansky 1999) (Siff 2003)

We will briefly define these tensions for the reader's awareness and, hopefully, to gain understanding of application if warranted. All these definitions of muscle tension are taken directly from the book *Supertraining* in 2003.

Acyclic describes speed movements involving rapid changes in position of the entire body or its links. The type of tension produced is a quick, momentary muscular contraction (i.e., boxing punch). However, a repetition of actions at a specific fast tempo (i.e., sprinting) would be an example of cyclic tension. Acyclic movements are distinguished by brief episodes of powerful muscular work and cyclic movements by the maintenance of optimal power for a relatively long time. Tonic muscular tension is characterized by significant and relatively prolonged muscle contraction. The speed with which it is developed, however, does not have major significance. This type of tension may be observed in wrestling when one athlete pins another to the mat, in weightlifting when the lifter holds a barbell overhead, and in many highly controlled gymnastic maneuvers. In all these cases, the muscles are working at the limit of their force capabilities. However, tonic tension can be of a much smaller magnitude when it is necessary to hold a pose (e.g., pistol shooting or gymnastics). Depending upon the type of sport, the characteristics of the strength displayed by tonic tension are determined by strength-endurance or absolute strength. (Siff 2003)

It also is important that it is proven that as absolute strength increases, then strength endurance also increases in a linear manner.

Phasic tension refers to dynamic muscular work in exercises requiring production of a driving force of a given magnitude. Such exercises are very frequently cyclic movements where each cycle has its own changing rhythm of muscular contraction, relaxation, and frequency of repetition. Here the speed with which maximal motor force is developed is not so important but strength or speed-strength endurance play a vital role. The type of exercise, the magnitude of tension (i.e., rowing), the temp of cyclic movement (e.g., swimming or speed skating), or both tempo and tension (i.e., cycling) can have major effects on how the muscles work. It is also possible to develop the ability to carry out phasic work of long duration at moderate tension (e.g., distance running and swimming). (Siff 2003)

Phasic-tonic tension occurs when dynamic work changes to stabilization or when stabilization changes to movement as a result of different rhythms or tempos of activity (gymnastics, judo, wrestling, ballet, etc.). The qualitative aspects of strength preparation in these cases are very complex and multifaceted. One type of sport or even one sport exercise may require both tonic and phasic tension involving a rapid transition from one type of tension to another at a high intensity of effort in each of them. This occurs in gymnastics during the switch from the dynamic to the static or stabilization elements or when a boxer quickly attacks resistance imposed by his opponents. (Siff 2003)

Explosive force is inherent to the following types of muscular tension: explosive-isometric, explosive-ballistic, and explosive-reactive-ballistic. Explosive-isometric tension is inherent to movements in which significant resistance is overcome (e.g., snatching or jerking a barbell, some elements in gymnastics and wrestling, or throwing a heavy projectile). A basic characteristic of these movements is the need to develop a large working force whose maximum is achieved isometrically at the end of the movement. This type of tension also occurs in plyometric activities during the brief transition phase between rapid eccentric and concentric contraction. (Siff 2003)

This important science, unfortunately, has created (due to individual perceptions/bias) an avenue for completely ignorant sport coaches (unfortunately, even many physical educators in public schools and professors in our hallowed universities) to claim they know how to train/teach their kids to be explosive using body weight and little coaching complexities (e.g., it is much harder to teach a large volume of people how to clean and jerk than it is to jump on a box). This has led to a whole train wreck in what the general population perceives is training for performance (e.g., cardiovascular doctrine, Western periodization, CrossFit, walking ten thousand steps a day will make you healthy, etc.). The ridiculous use and overtraining that has come out of the simple bodyweight plyometrics has allowed all aspects of people to think they know what great training is, and this is totally false as usual. Sport coaches are not strength coaches. They need to stick to coaching their sport in the Xs and Os and not pretend that they know or understand how to train the human body. Program design for training all aspects of the human population is very important, and I learned that from the best strength and conditioning coach in the country in his time, and Force 46 still knows and believes he is the best in all aspects still to this day! Even though Coach has passed, I have not forgotten all that he did and just have moved some aspects forward.

The diversity of the conditions under which muscles work in sport is responsible for the differences in motor activity and, consequently, the development of a specific strength capability. Categorization of strength capabilities into four discrete types (absolute strength, speed-strength, explosive strength and strength-endurance) can be somewhat restrictive, because all of them are interrelated in their production and development despite their inherent specificity. They are rarely, if ever, displayed separately but are the components of every movement. The strength ability most characteristic of sporting activities is explosive strength as displayed in acyclic and cyclic movements. If attention is paid to strength or speed-strength (depending upon external conditions), then the two general abilities, namely explosive strength and strength-endurance, are the basis for the production of all sporting movements. (Siff 2003)

With respect to physical education, Siff has already stated that the essence of sport is human movement, so physical education programs should emphasize movement every day in class. The myth that has been created in the United States is that "physical education is not for athletes, it is for the nonathletes." This is an entirely ignorant and wrong belief. Human movement is the essence of sport as well as the essence in life for all people no matter what your personal pursuit in life is!

Explosive-ballistic tension is characteristic of movements in which maximal force is applied against a relatively small resistance (e.g., shot put, javelin, baseball, or the serve in tennis). Here the motive force reaches a maximum quickly in the beginning and middle ranges of the movement, then begins to diminish. Due to inertia and muscular force (which at the end of the working amplitude does not exceed the weight of the load), the load has no acceleration but is only maintaining its existing velocity. As the resistance increases, this type of muscular tension changes to explosive-isometric. A ballistic movement may be preceded in its concentric working phase by muscle stretch. (Siff 2003)

Explosive-reactive-ballistic tension has the same characteristics as the explosive-ballistic type except for the regime of muscular work.

> Here the preliminary stretch phase is sharp and pronounced, after which there is an immediate change to concentric work. This can be observed in some throwing events and during individual elements of wrestling, gymnastics, figure skating, volleyball, tennis, or kicking a football. (Siff 2003)

Siff and Verkhoshansky went on to eloquently describe parameters and importance in flexibility. "Regular exercise that involves the full range of joint motion generally enhances flexibility" (Siff 2003). Zatsiorsky, 1995 states that athletes tend to develop patterns of flexibility which are characteristic of their particular sport. This clearly demonstrates the reason why specificity applies very little for young multisport athletes, and if the number one goal for strength and conditioning is injury prevention, then coaches need to look far beyond specificity. A lifting study from the *1984 Weightlifting Yearbook* speaks directly to the echo chamber for sport specific training.

> Over a period of years, they studied (at the Voronezhesky Farming Institute) the influence of kettlebell lifting on the development of fundamental physical qualities. Based on the results of the first control tests, 1,000 M cross-country, 100 M run, pull-ups, standing long jump. Three study groups were formed from the students who took part. Two experimental (19 men) and one control (21 men) of equivalent capabilities. (*1984 Weightlifting Yearbook*)

> The control group trained in the specific tests, and the two experimental groups trained with kettlebells. The results of the experimental groups were higher than those of the control group in all of the tests. (*The Russian Kettlbell Challenge*, Tsattsouline 2001)

> This demonstrates that kettlebell training is an effective means of physical education that develops basic physical qualities and increases physical work capacity. (*1984 Weightlifting Yearbook*)

This also demonstrates that the idea of training specific to a particular sport or tests is not necessarily the most effective way to improve or reach one's potential.

When looking at the results of this study, the Soviet scientists could not explain the spectacular all-around fitness gains from the standpoint of specificity but were too practical to be fzsed by this mystery. "Understanding is a delaying tactic (as a novelist put it). Do you want to understand how to swim or do you want to jump in and start swimming? Only people who are afraid of the water want to understand, other people jump in and get wet" (Tsatsouline 2001).

> It is known that if physical exercise lacks two fundamental qualities (accessibility and effectiveness), it loses its value as a means of physical education. Accessibility implies the following: the technique of the exercise is sufficiently simple; the exercise offers the ability to train individually or in groups; the simplicity of the training equipment; the training equipment provides the least chance of injury; the equipment allows a wide age range among the participants. The value of a means of physical education grows considerably if it can be utilized by different age groups and ability levels. It is also important to note that one must train periodically with an experienced coach controlling the training plan. (*1984 Weightlifting Yearbook*)

This highlights the problems we are seeing in the coaching realm in public schools and at the youth levels specifically. This also happens with many of the small colleges where if they actually have hired a strength and conditioning coach, the programs and training facilities are a major disappointment to say the least. The force 46 barrel was developed with much of this science in mind, and that is why I have been training with it for the past twenty years and counting as well as training a wide age range with this great implement (ages ten to seventy-two, both male and female).

The massive preoccupation of Western gym users with fixed bicycles or treadmill jogging to promote cardiovascular conditioning may then be seen to be potentially detrimental to serious athletes whose joints need to operate over a far more expansive range. These same scientists also discourage conventional push-ups and sit-ups because they tend to limit the functional range of motion of the shoulder and trunk regions respectively. It should be noted, however, that moderate intensity treadmill training of rats produces neither muscle hypertrophy nor increased growth of intramuscular connective tissue. Prolonged low-intensity training evidently can increase the cardiovascular system but not the musculoskeletal system. (Siff 2003)

Apparently, it is anaerobic, muscle endurance training which has the most pronounced effect on enhancing the concentration and strength of collagenous tissue and its junction zones. In contrast to chronic training, single exercise sessions, occasional stretching, or sprint training do not produce significant increase in junction strength, although sprinting produces marked increases in ligament mass and concentration. (Tipton et al. 1974). Just as ligaments become stronger and stiffer when subjected to increased stress, so they become weaker and less stiff with decreased stress, immobilization, and inactivity" (Tipton et al. 1970). Practical experience has led to recognition for four fairly traditional categories of stretching, namely static, ballistic, passive, and contract-relax (or PNF-proprioceptive neuromuscular facilitation) stretching. To this list may be added normal, full range of movement exercise, since it also tends to increase both active and passive flexibility. In addition, Olympic weightlifters are among the supplest of all athletes despite beliefs to the contrary" (Siff 1987). Furthermore, a combination of stretching and weight training exercises as a supplement to a sprint training program produces significantly greater increases in speed over an unsupplemented sprint program" (Siff 1987, in Siff 2003).

A large difference between active and passive flexibility (a measure which we may call the flexibility deficit FD) correlates strongly with the incidence of soft tissue injury. The flexibility deficit decreases significantly by means of the concurrent use of stretching and resistance training particularly if strength exercises are performed in the zone of active flexibility deficiency. Flexibility training should always be combined with neuromuscular training to produce efficient functional range of motion. Contract-relax, hold-relax, and other PNF methods use the different stretch reflexes to promote muscle relaxation. Sudden unloading, the sudden removal of external resistance imposed under strong isometric or dynamic conditions (e.g., the end of the jerk, completion of a heavy squat or bench press, throwing a shot or medicine ball, short bursts of strong electro muscular contraction). It has been shown that this means produces the greatest relaxation response of all the means currently used. You should always remember that the fundamental purpose of stretching is to enhance performance and reduce the likelihood of injury. (Siff 2003)

The other major point to citing some of this research is that it is clear that multi-joint movements in strength training is essential to training athletes, and far too often, the prevailing perception in sports especially in youth and high school is the sport coach (who is not an actual strength coach) starts trying to implement seriously flawed training protocols under the guise of sport specific training, and things quickly get out of hand. I have watched this for literally my entire life, and things seem to be getting worse, which is truly hard to believe.

[*Supertraining* does a great job discussing the limitations of anatomical movement analysis. This information is especially important to point out.] "Standard anatomical textbook approaches describing the action of certain muscle groups in controlling isolated joint actions such as flexion, extension, and rotation frequently are used to identify which muscles should be trained to enhance performance in sport. Virtually, every bodybuilding and sports training publication invokes this approach in describing how a given exercise or machine "works" a given muscle group. Most of the clinical texts on muscle testing and rehabilitation also follow this script. The appropriateness of this tradition, however, recently has been questioned on the basis of biomechanical analysis of multi-articular joint actions. (Zajac and Gordon 1989; *Supertraining* 1999; and Siff 2003)

This type of classical method of functional anatomy defines a given muscle, for instance, as a flexor or extensor on the basis of the torque that it produces around a single joint. The reality is that the nature of the body as a linked system of many joints means that muscles that do not span other joints can still produce acceleration about those joints. Mechanical systems of the body are nonlinear. There is no simple relationship between velocity, angle, and torque about a single joint in a complex sporting movement. Also, to this point, a single muscle group can simultaneously perform several different stabilizing and moving actions about one joint. There also is a fundamental difference between the dynamics of single and multiple joint movements. Forces on one segment can be caused by motion of other segments. Uniarticular muscles or even biarticular muscles (like the biceps or triceps), where only one of the joints is constrained to move, the standard approach is acceptable but not if several joints are free to move concurrently. Obviously, normal human movement in daily work and sport significantly is related to the mechanical systems approach rather than the tradition of the anatomical approach. The fact that muscles certainly do act to accelerate all joints has profound implications for the analysis of movement. For instance, muscles that cross the ankle joint can extend and flex the knee joint much more than they do the ankle. Biomechanical analysis reveals that multiarticular muscles may even accelerate a spanned joint in a direction opposite to that of the joint to which it is applying torque. In the apparently simple action of standing, the soleus, usually labeled as an extensor of the ankle, accelerates the knee (which it does not span) into extension twice as much as it acts to accelerate the ankle (which it does span) into extension for positions near upright posture. (Zajac and Gordon 1989; *Supertraining* 1999; and Siff 2003)

A piece of research that goes along with our program design is strengthening threshold.

> The development of strength requires that the intensity of the stimulus be gradually increased. It was discovered that every stimulus has a specific *strengthening threshold*, the achievement of which fails to elicit any further increase in muscular strength (Muller 1962). The less trained the muscles are [i.e., beginners/novice], the further the strengthening threshold from the initial [untrained] state. The rate at which strength increases from the initial level to the strengthening threshold expressed as a percentage of the current maximum strength, is independent of sex, age, muscle group and the level of the strengthening threshold (Muller 1962). After the strengthening threshold has been reached, strength can be increased only by intensifying the training (e.g., substituting stronger means, devising more effective combinations, or increasing the volume of work). (Siff 2003)

This is another reason why we created the force 46 barrels. There is a real problem with sport coaches overtraining athletes in their sport and then having the kids engage in high-volume training modes such as plyometrics, long-distance running, inappropriate lifting, or other highly publicized drills. The overuse and overtraining becomes difficult to stomach, and yet this is going to another level with the NIL and current "me" society that is looking to get noticed in all aspects of life.

A final section of important science dealing with developing athletes deals with what Siff calls the structure of motor abilities and physical fitness for movement.

> It has been established that, concurrent with the change in the factor composition (and, consequently, the motor abilities that determine sporting success), there is a definite overestimation of their significance as proficiency grows. One of them displays a greater significance while another becomes less important (e.g., there is a general tendency in speed-strength sports for muscular strength to decrease and the ability to produce explosive force to increase). However, there is an exception in weightlifters because they experience a sharp increase in relative strength with growth in proficiency. The fitness factor proportion of the individual motor abilities such as absolute strength, starting strength, and acceleration strength changes concurrently with growth in proficiency. That is the degree of correlation of proficiency with the given factor. This clearly corroborates the abovementioned decreasing role of absolute strength activities in enhancing speed-strength.
>
> Research also shows that the most important changes in the composition and structure of physical fitness occur primarily during the beginning stage of training. At the high sports mastery level, significant changes in the structure of physical fitness do not occur, thereby emphasizing the stability of the advanced neuromotor programs and contributions by the individual fitness factor. (Siff 2003)

This information is important because what I have observed with sport coaches over the last thirty years is that they watch too much TV. Specifically, they watch their favorite division I level team or professional team. Or they read some article about how their favorite athlete trains; and they try and pass that on to the elementary, middle school, or high school athlete. This, in turn, completely misses on how to appropriately develop the athlete. Not to mention the fact that the sport coaches are not strength coaches.

As stated earlier, the overtraining from poorly trained personal trainers, sport coaches, etc. has made a mockery out of fitness training and culminates in nothing but mediocrity and the next wave of future parents who have no clue about sporting movement, weight loss, and fitness. I am sure Coach Stucky understood this bit of information because his program design is still the best for all levels of training in my opinion.

The role of specific abilities, nonspecific abilities, and leveling motor abilities are also something to pay attention to.

The levelling abilities ensure the effective development of the key motor ability, which expresses the motor requirements of the specific sporting action. The levelling abilities balance out and smooth the interaction between all other abilities. The role of specific is to secure the productivity of the key motor abilities. The role of nonspecific ability becomes apparent where the specific ability is displayed under difficult conditions. For example, if speed of movement (the specific ability) is the primary requirement but displaying it to a high level is difficult because of external resistance, then muscular strength (the nonspecific ability) acts as an assisting factor. On the other hand, if the level of explosive strength decreases due to increasing fatigue, for example, then the required motor effect can be maintained by special endurance processes. Research and practical experience indicate that the formation and development of specific motor abilities is not based upon the synthesis of the motor abilities developed individually or the gradual transformation of some abilities into others. Instead, motor abilities retain their separate characteristics and a specific neuromotor program is established by rational training, which integrates the contributions of other motor abilities. (Siff 2003)

Once again, I believe Coach Stucky's program design addressed much of this research.

"Rosenzweig (1984) concluded that the capacity for plastic neural changes is present not only early in life but throughout most or all of one's life span. These changes become particularly evident if one is exposed to a sufficiently enriched environment providing novel, complex, and cognitively challenging stimulation, a finding which stresses the importance of not limiting one's training to simple, largely unchallenging repetitive patterns of training with exactly the same weights or machines. This is one reason why it may be important to employ variations utilizing numerous different means, methods, and exercises that draw on integrative whole-body disciplines such as physiotherapeutic PNF (proprioceptive neuromuscular facilitation)" (Siff 2003). This also is Coach Stucky and a clear reason for the force 46 barrel.

The working effect of a sporting movement is simply the result of the specific form of organization and control of one's interaction with the environment. However, the fundamental concept of sports technique appears not merely as the organization of the motor components of the sporting movement. Rather, it is the athlete's ability to manage the external conditions competently and exploit the possibilities that they offer.

Sports technique is not a constant that can be achieved once, but it is the result of continued progress from a lower to a higher level of perfection. (Verkhoshansky 1977 and *Supertraining* 1999). Therefore, the ability to achieve one's real potential in specific motor tasks by maintaining a particular system of movement is the essence of sporting proficiency. Continual improvement in this ability is fundamental to the training process, and the degree to which motor potential is realized is the criterion of its effectiveness. (Siff 2003)

All these speaks to how Coach Stucky developed athletes, movement, and created an environment where all people can be successful if they want to work for it. It is one thing to read information, and it is another thing to be able to apply the information to create new results in programming philosophy. Coach Stucky was way ahead of his time, and that allowed force 46 and the force 46 barrels to be ahead of its time along with our program design in the weight room and physical education classes. The following science is more of what Coach Stucky was cognizant about, and in later years, I researched on my own and smiled because reading something is one thing and actually living and performing it is another, and that is when expertise occurs.

The following cited science comes from the book *Science and Practice of Strength Training*. The book was written by Vladimir Zatsiorsky.

Adaptation as a Main Law of Training

If a training routine is planned and executed correctly, the result of systematic exercise is improvement of physical fitness, particularly strength, as the body adapts to physical load. In a broad sense, the word *adaptation* means the adjustment of an organism to its environment. If the environment changes, the organism changes to better survive in these new conditions. In biology, adaptation is considered one of the main features of living species. Exercise or regular physical work is a very powerful stimulus for adaptation. The major objective in training is to induce specific adaptations to improve performance results. This requires adherence to a carefully planned and executed training program. From the practical point of view, the following four features of the adaptation process assume primary importance for training:

The stimulus magnitude (overload)
Accommodation

Specificity
Individualization

Training loads can be roughly classified according to their magnitude as:

Stimulating—the magnitude of the training load is above the neutral level, and positive adaptation may take place.

Retaining—the magnitude is in the neutral zone at which the level of fitness is maintained.

Detraining—the magnitude of the load leads to a decrease in performance results in the functional capabilities of the individual or both. (Zatsiorsky 1995).

Accommodation

If the individual employs the same exercise with the same training load over a long period of time, performance gains decrease. This is a manifestation of the biological law of accommodation, often considered a general law of biology. According to this law, the response of a biological object to a given constant stimulus decreases over time. By definition, accommodation is the decrease in response of a biological object to a continued stimulus. In training, the stimulus is physical exercise. Because of accommodation, it is inefficient to use standard exercises or a standard training load over a long period of time. Training programs must vary.

To avoid or decrease the negative influence of accommodation, training programs are periodically modified. In principle, there are two ways to modify training programs:

Quantitative-changing training loads (for instance, the total amount of weight lifted)
Qualitative-replacing the exercises

Qualitative changes are very broadly used in the training of elite athletes, at least by the most creative. (Zatsiorsky 1995)

Individualization

All people are different. The same exercises or training methods elicit a greater or smaller effect in various individuals. Innumerable attempts to mimic the training routines of famous athletes have proven unsuccessful. Only the general ideas underlying noteworthy training programs, not the entire training protocol, should be understood and creatively employed. The same holds true for average values derived from training practices and scientific research. (Zatsiorsky 1995)

Mechanical Feedback

All strength exercises, depending on the type of resistance, can be separated into those with and those without mechanical feedback. Consider, for instance, a paddling movement in water. In hydrodynamics, the force applied to water is proportional to the velocity squared ($F = kV^2$). However, the oar's velocity is the result of an individual's efforts, an external muscular force. Here active muscular force leads to higher oar velocity, which in turn increases water resistance. Then to overcome the increased water resistance, the muscle force is elevated. Thus, increased water resistance can be regarded as an effect of the high muscular force (mechanical feedback). Sports movements usually involve mechanical feedback: the movement, as well as resistance, is changed as a result of an individual's force application. Mechanical feedback is absent only in the performance of isometric exercises and in work with isokinetic devices.

Strength values at the weakest positions (the so-called sticking points) are also very important.

The heaviest weight that is lifted through a full range of joint motion cannot be greater than the strength of the weakest point. This weight taxes only a certain percentage of the maximum force at other joint angles. Many consider this a disadvantage of exercises using free weights. Special cams of variable radii are used in some strength training devices to provide maximal or at least near-maximal muscular tension throughout the full range of joint motion. This is achieved by changing the moment arm of the machine so that the resistance, in turn, varies. Three different approaches have been developed to maximize the training benefit of resistance work. In the first, maximal force is developed in the weakest body position (termed the peak-contraction principle). In the second approach, near-maximal force is attained throughout the complete range of joint motion (accommodating resistance [i.e., chains]). In the third, exercises are constructed to develop maximal force at the precise angular position in which maximal efforts are developed during the main movement. This third approach is called the accentuation of muscular efforts. (Zatsiorsky 1995)

Neural (Central) Factors

The central nervous system (CNS) is of paramount importance in the exertion and development of muscular strength. Muscular strength is determined not only by the quantity of involved muscle mass but also by the extent to which individual fibers in a muscle are voluntarily activated (by intramuscular coordination). Maximal force exertion is a skilled act in which many muscles must be appropriately activated. This coordinated activation of many muscle groups is called intermuscular coordination. As a result of neural adaptation, superior athletes can better coordinate the activation of fibers in single muscles and in muscle groups. In other words, they have better intramuscular and intermuscular coordination.

The recruitment order of MUs is relatively fixed for a muscle involved in a specific motion even if the movement velocity or rate of force development alters. However, the recruitment order can be changed if the multifunction muscle operates in different motions. Different sets of MUs within one muscle might have a low threshold for one motion and a high threshold for another. The variation in recruitment order is partially responsible for the specificity of training effect in heavy resistance exercise. If the objective in training is the full development of a muscle (not high athletic performance), one must exercise this muscle in all possible ranges of motion. (Zatsiorsky 1995)

Intermuscular Coordination

Every exercise, even the simplest one, is a skilled act requiring the complex coordination of numerous muscle groups. The entire movement pattern, rather than the strength of single muscles or the movement of single joints, must be the primary training objective. Thus, an athlete should use one joint and only as a supplement to the main training program. Athletes in sports such as rowing or weight lifting that require the simultaneous bilateral contraction of the same muscle groups should use similar exercises to eliminate bilateral deficits. However, the elite super heavy lifters employ exercises such as stepping up on a bench with barbells 180 kg and heavier (unilateral). They do this to avoid the extremely high loading that occurs during squatting exercises in which the barbell weight can exceed 350 kg. In the case of the bottleneck effect, when low strength in one joint of a kinematic chain limits performance (e.g., knee extensor strength is the limiting factor in squatting), the coach should first try to change the exercise to redistribute the load among different muscle groups. Only after that is an isolated knee extension against a resistance advisable. The important limitation of many strength training machines is that they are designed to train muscles, not movement. Because of this, they are not the most important training tool for athletes. (Zatsiorsky 1995)

The Peak-Contraction Principle

Historically, the peak-contraction approach is the oldest one. The idea is to focus efforts on increasing muscle strength primarily at the weakest points of the human strength curve. In practice, the peak-contraction principle is realized in one of three ways:

Selection of a proper body position. The resistance offered by the lifted load is not, in reality, constant over a full range of joint motion. The resistance is determined by the moment of gravitational force (i.e., by the product of weight and horizontal distance to the axis of rotation) rather than by the weight of the implement or the body part itself. The moment of gravitational force is maximal when the center of gravity of the lifted load is on the same horizontal line as the axis of rotation. In this case, the lever arm of the gravitational force is greatest. By varying body posture, it is possible to an extent to superimpose the human strength curve on the resistance curve in a desirable manner. The peak-contraction principle is realized, if "worst comes to worst," when the external resistance (moment of gravity force) is maximal at the point where muscular strength is minimal.

Use of special training devices. Many times, machines are developed to try to be applicable to strength issues but end up being of limited use in reality (i.e., smith machine). The arm curl is one that had been developed to create the maximal resistance coinciding with the weakest point on the human strength curve. If a barbell was used in the arm curl, the maximal resistance would be at the horizontal position of the forearms (ninety degrees). In contrast to the situation with the peak-contraction principle, the strength of forearm flexion at the elbow joint is maximal, not minimal, at this position. The created machine/implement places the highest resistance at the top of the bicep curl.

Slow beginning motion. A slow start can be used in strength drills such as the inverse curl. The maximal resistance in this exercise is offered while the trunk is in the horizontal position. If the movement begins too fast, the lift in the intermediate range of motion is performed at the expense of the kinetic energy acquired in the first part of the movement. The erector spinae muscles then are not fully activated. Experienced athletes and coaches advocate a slow start for this drill. (Zatsiorsky 1995)

Accommodating Resistance

The main idea of accommodating resistance is to develop maximal tension throughout the complete range of motion rather than at a particular (e.g., weakest point). This can be achieved in two ways. One type of system offers high resistance without mechanical feedback. In this case, the speed of motion is constant no matter how much force is developed. This principle is realized in isokinetic equipment. The movement speed on such devices can be preset and maintained (kept constant) during a motion regardless of the amount of force applied against the machine. The working muscles are maximally loaded throughout the complete range of motion. (Zatsiorsky 1995)

Another type of system provides variable resistance that is accommodated to either the human strength curve or movement speed. In some machines, resistance is applied in concert with the human strength curve (Nautilus-type equipment). Because of the special odd-shaped cams on these machines, the lever arm of the resistance force or applied force is variable so that the load varies accordingly. (Zatsiorsky 1995).

Another type of exercise apparatus accommodates resistance to movement velocity. The higher the velocity, the greater the resistance offered by the system. These devices are typically based on hydraulic principles. The velocity of movements with hydraulic machines, in contrast to isokinetic devices, may vary depending on the strength of the trainee.

Scientific experts have often questioned the validity of claims for high exercise efficiency with accommodating resistance. Exercises performed with strength training machines are biomechanically different from natural movements and traditional exercises. Most notably, the number of degrees of freedom (permissible movement directions) is limited from six in natural movements to only one with exercise machines. The typical acceleration-deceleration pattern is also different. Though isokinetic training may have certain advantages in clinical rehabilitation settings, studies have repeatedly failed to demonstrate that accommodating resistance exercises (e.g., isotonic, variable cams) hold an advantage over free weight exercises for increasing muscular strength and inducing muscle hypertrophy. (Zatsiorsky 1995)

All the science and information presented at this point led to the creation of the force 46 barrel. I was giving a community presentation at the high school I worked at in 2003. After I completed my presentation, a father came up to me and said how impressed he was with the information given. He also stated that he knew in ten minutes that I knew what I was talking about, and he was really glad I was coaching his son. This positive feedback then led to me creating an adult strength and conditioning class on Saturday mornings for parents. I also knew that Jerry Prenatt was the owner of a foundry that produced many steel products, molds, castings, etc. Jerry was a very successful and self-employed businessman with great character and caring for quality.

Some of the top strength and conditioning professionals were engaging in keg lifting and its benefits. I also liked the concept but felt the kegs were too limited for what I was looking for overall. Also the politics in society and lack of common sense made me realize that some hypocrites might deem keg lifting as promoting drinking, so this plus that limited range of motion made me think of talking with Jerry. I spoke to Jerry about my beliefs in program design and inquired if he would be able to build me an implement that elicited the benefits of keg lifting but could mimic all the power lifts and weightlifting lifts I feel should be primary in any great strength and conditioning program. I envisioned this implementation to be useful in all aspects of a daily program and also could stand alone on some lifting days if need be.

Jerry came up with some prototypes, and it was exactly what I was looking for. Jerry got the patents, and I began implementing the philosophy of how to use the barrels and many possibilities and reasoning in the scope of program design. Unfortunately, my life was occupied with being a teacher, coach, and then father, so we basically kept the concept our own secret, and I continued training athletes with them, but that was as far as we went at that time. Things changed dramatically when I decided to leave teaching to start my own strength and conditioning business. We began scientific testing and have more studies to come in the coming years and now trademarked our concept as the force 46 barrel.

This great science is presented throughout the book because any individual who wants to train another really should know and understand this scientific information. None of these great books with real science were ever put in college curriculums, and still, to this day, they are not. We, as a country, keep teaching our own versions of fitness and junk science that is why we see all the nonsense in sport training, weight loss, and overall fitness. It becomes a game or competition or see who can lift the most weight. A great training program can accomplish all these elements. Chasing a one-thousand-pound dead lift is fine, but that is not the answer to great fitness and health, nor is it the answer to great sport or movement performance. I would much rather be Bruce Lee than having the goal of who can have the biggest bicep.

A perfect example to what I am talking about was a very talented player at the University of Arkansas. This player was likely the best athlete I had ever seen at that time. He was 205 lbs., and he back squatted 660 lbs. raw, he bench-pressed 440 lbs., he ran a 4.5 forty-yard dash, and he vertical jumped forty-one inches in 1992. My point to this story is that he was "shredded." He was lean. If he wasn't a division I football player and actually had the goal of lifting for a powerlifting number all year round, then I am sure he could have pulled nine hundred plus pounds nondrug and legit. He was an absolute freak of nature, and he also trained under John Stucky… enough said! JD was a good friend of mine on the football team.

Political Culture in Public Schools

I happened to see a headline in the news from the World Economic Forum. The title of the article was "Our Education System Is Losing Relevance." Here's how to unleash its potential. I had an immediate thought that this was likely going to be the same rehash of old trash but also might have some very important points that are very true. I was correct in my initial thought. The article stated that education today is in crisis. The second line stated, "Even before the coronavirus pandemic struck, in many parts of the world, children who should be in school aren't" (Krishnan 2020). There is the status quo argument that has been said since the 1970s and 1980s. The big problem worldwide seems to always indicate that not enough children are in school. Ironically, that is not the issue in the United States. Our nation's kids are in school, and education is in an epic educational crisis on many levels. My wife and I have taught in the public schools with over fifty-five years of highly recognized experience, and the idea that kids aren't in school is the furthest thing from the problem (at least in the United States).

Educational leaders have known for many years (at least by the time "No Child Left Behind" and likely years previous to this train wreck) that the industrialized model that is the United States education system is completely wrong and irrelevant. IQ means little, and memorizing bureaucratic-driven information is far from indicating whether a human being is smart. Education can't seem to correct the problem mainly because as G. K. Chesterton stated, "It isn't that they can't see the solution. It is that they can't see the problem." When the bureaucracy can't see the problem and the proprietary programming and political corruption takes hold, then the change that these entities shout about becomes chasing their tails over the same rehash of old trash, and nothing really changes but a creation of more problems.

As we will describe in this chapter (with relations to schools), it's not about children not being in class, it is about all the problems of what and how things are taught in classes and then a whole lot more. The article did state some real truths.

> Workers with a relatively fixed set of skills and knowledge are losing their relevance in an era of innovation, disruption, and constant change where adaptability and learning agility are most needed. Sixty percent of future jobs haven't been developed yet, and 40 percent of nursery-age children (kindergarteners) in schools today will need to be self-employed to have any form of income (WEF Future of Jobs Report). We need to prepare students for jobs that haven't been created yet and to become entrepreneurs. (Krishnan 2020)

What we need to learn, how we learn, and the role of the teacher are all changing. These are very true and real statements. The simple fact is that the education system needs a complete overhaul. We do not need children to take four years of English language arts when it can be taught properly in a semester at the high school level. We do not need to take multiple years of algebra and geometry because it can be taught in a semester properly. Differentiated instruction allows for individual students who may need more higher level practice (like an airline pilot) to get the high level geometry instruction without wasting three years or more to do it.

An intelligent person would have to ask some telling questions as well like, Why are our students working on English and writing for twelve years and somehow all college students need to take some form of English? How can students have taken literally twelve years of English / writing / American literature / poetry for their K-12 years and somehow not have the skills yet? If this is somehow true, then, clearly, twelve years of public education has failed miserably, and yet our experts can't figure out why education is failing? They see the solution but do not see the problem! These points are extremely important because the very people who lay claim to improving the plight of education and world issues keep using the same language: "transform education," "access," "equity," "impact," "reset education," "sustainable goals," "economic independence," etc. The words do not mean anything, and they definitely do not mean change. They see the solution, but they do not see the problem!

I found another article in the news written by Pamela Burdman from the *Scientific American*. The title of the article is "To Keep Students in STEM Field, Let's Weed Out the Weed-Out Math Classes."

> All routes to STEM degrees run through calculus classes. Each year, hundreds of thousands of college students take introductory calculus. Only a fraction ultimately complete a STEM degree, and research about why students abandon such degrees suggests that traditional calculus courses are one of the reasons. With scientific understanding and innovation increasingly central to solving twenty-first-century problems, this loss of talent is something society can ill afford. (Burdman 2022)

This clearly shows that the educational problem is far more than kids not having access. It is more about the politics and status quo from the very people who claim to be educators.

Math departments alone are unlikely to solve this dilemma. Several of the promising calculus reforms highlighted in our report "Charting a New Course: Investigating Barriers on the Calculus Pathway to STEM" that was published with the California Education Learning Lab. This report was spearheaded by professors outside of math departments. It's time for STEM faculty to prioritize collaboration across disciplines to transform math classes from weed-out mechanisms to fertile terrain for cultivating a diverse generation of STEM researchers and professionals. This is uncharted territory.

In 2013, life sciences faculty at the University of California, Los Angeles, developed a two-course sequence that covers classic calculus topics such as the derivative and the integral but emphasizes their application in a biological context. The professors used modeling of complex systems such as biological and physiological processes as a framework for teaching linear algebra and a starting point for teaching the basics of computer programming to support students' use of systems of differential equations. Creating this course, mathematics for life scientists, wasn't easy. The life sciences faculty involved, none of whom had a joint appointment with the math department, said they resorted to designing the course themselves after math faculty rebuffed their overture. The math faculty feared creating a "watered down" course without a textbook (though after the course was developed, one math instructor taught some sections of the class). Besides math, the life sciences faculty said they experienced "significant pushback" from the chemistry and physics departments over concerns that the course wouldn't adequately prepare students for required courses in those disciplines. (Burdman 2022)

This is a perfect example of a specific problem in education. The politics, self-serving agendas, etc. from the very people who have educational titles and are supposed to be helping improve learning are actually the ones creating roadblocks and lessening advancement in their own fields. The article goes on to say the following:

According to recently published research led by UCLA education researchers, students in the new classes ended up with "significantly higher grades" in subsequent physics, chemistry, and life science courses than students in the traditional calculus course even when controlling for factors such as demographics, prior preparation, and math grades. Student's interest doubled according to surveys. The UCLA example highlights longstanding concerns about the relevance of traditional calculus for biology students. Traditionally, college math departments have overseen general education math courses for students in other majors.

A little over two decades ago, biology faculty, convened by the Mathematics Association of America, advocated that for biology majors, "statistics, modeling, and graphical representation should take priority" over calculus. But change has been slow until life science departments got involved. The article goes on to mention this movement from the life sciences as an important

> strategy for increasing persistence rates particu-
> larly among students traditionally excluded from
> STEM fields such as Black, Latino, and indige-
> nous students as well as women. (Burdman 2022)

I am sure this is true, but I wonder when we can get rid of all the race and gender stuff and just talk about all humans when it comes to improving education as a whole. I am Italian American, and I never even had actual physics, but physics makes sense to me because of strength and conditioning, and I learned it without having to go one hundred thousand dollars in debt from the above example, which is another point to understanding the problem and not just knowing the solution.

> Engineering departments also worry about calculus sequences driving attrition. Wright State University's solution also involved revising math offerings. But rather than changing the content of the calculus course, they focused on preparing students for calculus by emphasizing "engineer-ing motivation for math." In lieu of traditional calculus prerequisites such as precalculus or col-lege algebra, the engineering faculty launched a contextualized math course in 2004, emphasiz-ing problem-based learning. The course covers topics students need in sophomore engineering classes, including linear equations, quadratic equations, 2-D vectors, and complex numbers. A modest redesign of the engineering curriculum allows students to delay taking a traditional cal-culus sequence until later in their programs.

I can find fault here, however, it is not worth arguing their approach, and they made strides in improvement.

> Increasingly, leading math and science organizations are recognizing the importance of interdisciplinary collaboration. The MAA has a history of convening faculty from partner disciplines, and a *National Academies* 2013 publication called for reassessing math education in a cross-disciplinary context. The National Science Foundation, which funded both the UCLA and Wright State University innovations, recognizes the value of cross-disciplinary or 'convergence research,' which is driven by a compelling scientific or societal problem. Low persistence in STEM majors and lack of diversity in STEM fields are themselves pressing societal problems. (Burdman 2022)

Needless to say, this article is published in 2022, and the Wright State University solution appears to be addressed in 2004.

With all the talk about improving the plight of STEM, it should be easily interpreted that various political hoops must be jumped through just to get a sense of betterment in a train wreck of a status quo system. Not to mention that the big STEM push obviously trickled down to the public schools K-12, and as stated throughout this book, the implementation of the supposed importance was also done in a very political and poorly designed process, so any chance for improvement will be slim to none from most districts in the United States.

> [The article finishes with the classic circumstance.] Yet math departments without jointly-appointed professors seem to be less interested in evidence-based contributions from other disciplines to enhance the effectiveness of math

instruction or even aware of successes to date. The shift toward more practical applications of calculus is missing one key academic endorsement: publication in widely read journals, if the success of the courses is examined academically at all (Burdman 2022).

This is all addressed in our book in the first chapter with the follow the science echo chamber. We demonstrated the inefficiency of this with respect to the cardiovascular doctrine, yet the theme is inherent in almost every circumstance where education or solving problems or the simple idea of just improving and getting better is hindered!

Teaching in the public school system for twenty-five years has given me great insight in the very real problems in education. The complexity of politics and corruption has been fostered by many entities, and the standard operating procedures see no end in sight. There are many levels of corruption. There will be people who do not like or agree with the term corruption when it comes to education.

Let's take a look at this thought for a moment. There is a complex interconnected system within the public schools today. You must take into account that the school boards, administration, teachers and teachers union, local government, state government, and federal government are all involved. I was a young teacher when "No Child Left Behind" legislation was passed. This federal interference took the politics and corruption to new heights. It appears that hiding behind the guise of doing what is best for children would be prostituted and shaped by individual perceptions to push self-promoting agendas by all parties involved.

I learned in my masters of educational leadership that since before the ancient Egyptian times through to present day that the following statement is fact: "Any time a government tries to exert control, it leads to absolute corruption." This is easily the case in the present when talking about public schools. School boards, in my own experience, always have a number of members who push self-serving agendas to hang on to their position when, clearly, their agenda is not what is in the best interest of the kids. Many times, the makeup of the school board is such that it is near impossible to get a quality vote on any item due to the vastly political disparity within the board itself. This means, in short, there is a lot of wasted money and little gets done. The only thing that remains is the same discussion and arguments over what should be simple but ends up being the same rehash of the same trash.

The teacher unions, following their own outdated script and still following the industrialized mentality and model, love to push the narrative that everyone in the school system who has an opinion is equal. The reality is that systems thinking is corrupt by nature. The reality is that every teacher with a degree or certification is not equal, yet the schools want everyone to conform to this idea, so great ideas are diminished so others can save face and pretend they are import-ant. I remember dealing with this my entire career.

As far as fitness goes, that would be the cardiovascular doctrine, which scientifically was never true. I had a colleague that once stated, "I would never lift weights! I only do yoga!" It is fine that a so-called certified professional believes that yoga is the end-all. I have no prob-lem with any individual who enjoys doing yoga or any other type of exercise either. However, just because you personally like something does not mean that your preference will actually be the appropriate teaching knowledge, and yoga does not address what complete fit-ness actually is.

Ironically, this teacher, a couple years later, lost her job and went to jail for sleeping with a middle school student. It's a good thing that the public education echo chamber allowed her opinions to fester on yoga being the end-all as a form of teaching what is best for children and what is correct. This is why grading on the fitness factors is so important. Yoga is a beneficial form of exercise, however, it fails to sufficiently address all the fitness factors. The only exercise that truly addresses all fitness factors is strength and conditioning programmed in an appropriate manner and sequence that does not overtrain but improves all fitness factors consistently year after year. A great teacher would teach all the concepts of strength and conditioning and then lead students to choose other fitness activities in their weekly routine that addresses their likes and desires so they can have the ability to demonstrate actual fitness and not chase their tails as they get older. (Remember treadmills and walking ten thousand steps?)

"No Child Left Behind" along with the state government pushed the China theory to get teeth and support for their corrupt thought. The simple claim is that China is far ahead of the United States in education. I remember the national education leaders saying Chinese kids go to school 222 days a year and engage in a more rigorous curriculum, and that we have to change public schools to be able to stay ahead. This is the biggest lie and eerily similar to the cardiovascular doctrine. What have we achieved in reality with all this corrupt narrative? We have kids who hate school! We have state testing covering material that is for the most part irrelevant! We have high school kids in Pennsylvania take the Keystone exams in algebra and English language arts even though they already passed algebra and English language arts (somebody is getting rich off these tests and it isn't the students). We have a rigorous curriculum in geometry that has more vocabulary words to memorize than English language arts, and this somehow means that students are really smart? If public education was to even remotely be trying to help the kids, then they would realize that all the corruption needs to be abolished, and the schools need to stop teaching like it is 1920 industrialized education and proprietary programming.

Education needs to realize that with "No Child Left Behind," it has allowed itself to be further behind. School accountability brought us DIBELS testing. We actually test first graders to see if they can read forty-seven words per minute. I watched this absolutely destroy children's love of reading and instill fear that they can't read fast enough, and yet nothing gets done about this travesty. It is not important how fast a person reads, it is only important on what they comprehend and what they can do with the information as well as decipher whether the information is important or relevant.

I came across a Fox News article written by Joshua Q. Nelson in September 2022. The education department reported that reading scores dropped by the largest margin in more than thirty years. Marilyn Muller, a pro bono literacy advocate, told America's Newsroom that,

"Our daughter started kindergarten in a Massachusetts public school and very quickly showed signs that I now know are associated and linked with reading failure. She was frustrated by the task. She would avoid the task, and those behaviors would manifest with a refusal to go to school. In the afternoon, when she would get off the bus or I would pick her up at school, she would get into her safe space in the car and have what is basically called a meltdown after-school restraint."

This example is exactly what has happened in public schools everywhere, and it's the "No Child Left Behind" politics along with trying to push the China superiority in academics notion coupled with the state and federal testing that is causing decline in scores, stress in kids not enjoying school, and now the complete left socialist agenda. We actually have cases in schools where kids believe they are cats so they can dress up like a cat, kitty litter is provided for them at school, and they can even meow answers. This sentence alone could be a separate book on the current state of society and intelligence. Even worse, most of the testing has little to do with actually being smart or productive in society, so to continue to overtest on material that has little relevance to most school students and drive the false narrative that the last twenty years of government ill-advised thought that "No Child Left Behind" and the famous buzzwords like academic rigor and accountability has taken us to the point we are at now, and it is not good. (Hopefully, you see the analogy/trend of buzzwords in fitness and academics.)

The cardiovascular doctrine was never correct and yet prevailed in the United States for over sixty years. "No Child Left Behind" has been in place since George W. Bush was in office, and it is a total failure, yet our self-proclaimed experts sit around scratching their heads why irrelevant test scores are declining. "It is not that they cannot see the solution, it is that they cannot see the problem." This is where things get interesting, and the same echo chambers come out rehashing the same trash. Of course, COVID-19 is the new scapegoat. Yes, the handling of COVID-19 was a disaster, and our so-called experts and leaders dropped the ball in a big way, so they just need to look in the mirror and blame themselves. However, COVID-19 actually exposed the public school system as parents were able to actually see the ridiculous volume of busy work the students actually face on a day-to-day basis.

The epic failure did not just occur in the last two years with COVID-19. We have been blindly following "No Child Left Behind" for twenty years along with education's notorious quest for the next magic bullet (e.g. state test, national test, teachers biweekly test all on the same material mind you, inept curriculum directors who have little business driving school-wide curriculum and professional development, status quo school board and union practice, etc.), and that has led to the epic failure of testing and intelligence, not COVID-19. The political corruption that is education has caused the poor test scores, which we already have addressed.

I ran across an article written October 6, 2022, by Temple Grandin. The title of the article was "Against Algebra." Students need more exposure to the way everyday things work and are made. I knew without reading this article that it had to be echoing the same things I have been addressing in this chapter. After reading this article, Temple Grandin was absolutely correct and could easily take it much farther, which I think this chapter clearly does. Temple stated, "One of the most useless questions you can ask a kid is, What do you want to be when you grow up? The more useful question is, What are you good at? But schools aren't giving kids enough of a chance to find out."

The school district where I live has instituted a career readiness requirement that must be completed as it is a graduation requirement. Kids do not have to have all the answers as to what they want to be and do by the time they are eighteen. The vast majority of people will say they know and go to college, take on huge debt, then, lo and behold, start a completely different career that has nothing to do with what they went to college for. Ironically, the student debt still stays with them except for the current lucky few because our current president has allowed some students to apply to have their student debt eliminated, which is truly epic stupidity from any individual charged with making appropriate decisions for the people. Of course, you know, it will be the taxpayers who will be making up the difference for this little charade by an elected official.

Temple is a visual thinker who has autism, and she often thinks about how education fails to meet the needs of our very diverse minds. "We are shunting students into a one-size-fits-all curriculum instead of nurturing the budding builders, engineers, and inventors that our country needs." Actually, the way public education has been is actually shunting all aspects, and even the individuals who don't make waves and just follow the rules often become the very professionals who provide little in any kind of human advancement (e.g., cardiovascular doctrine). The point is if a person memorizes incorrect information because some political entity pushes a series of proprietary programming, then the person ends up considered intelligent, however, it is intelligence with incorrect knowledge. One would then have to conclude that this intelligent person is actually ignorant, and that is very much fact and the truth!

Temple went on to cite "No Child Left Behind" as a major culprit that echoes what I have stated as well. Nikhil Goyal in his book, *Schools on Trial: How Freedom and Creativity Can Fix Our Educational Malpractice*, illustrated that a new philosophy had supplanted hands-on learning for teaching to the test otherwise known as "drill, kill, bubble fill." Temple cited an article written a decade ago by Andrew Hacker titled "Is Algebra Necessary?" Hacker rebuked the insistence on algebra in schools, pointing out that the math taught in school was nothing like the math people use in their jobs. "Making mathematics mandatory" wrote Hacker, "prevents us from discovering and developing young talent. In the interest of maintaining rigor, we are actually depleting our pool of brainpower."

Temple went on to state:

> The irony has never been lost on me. I teach veterinarians, but I couldn't get into veterinary school myself because I couldn't do the math. In college, I had to drop a physics and a biomedical-engineering course. This screened me out of veterinary school and engineering. I had

to choose majors with lower math requirements, such as psychology and animal science, and I got tutoring to help me through. Today, even those doors would likely be closed to me because those degrees now have even higher math requirements. I recently received an email from a student who informed me that he had to take calculus for his undergraduate biology major. Biology was my favorite subject, but I would never have gotten past that barrier.

Ironically, I present much biological science in the barrel chapter that is applied to strength and conditioning, but I promise you whenever I had biology in high school, we never were taught to apply much of anything with respect to the corrupt script of curriculum, so I actually studied on my own for appropriate understanding and not worrying about whether I filled a correct bubble on a test.

A final thought Temple finishes with was, "Not only has our approach failed to help kids find their way in the world, but it also hasn't even improved their academic performance. By 2017, two-thirds of community-college students and one-third of four-year college students needed remedial math. But maybe the decline in performance points to a deficiency not so much in how well students master material but in what we are asking them to master." Temple was correct, so to make a final quick statement on this, I have two algebraic concepts in this book and a bunch of biological laws in my book that does not take 360 days (two years of high school) to learn, and I also did not even need a teacher to help me learn and apply the information. Everything about schools needs to change, and the government needs to be removed from the process or the corruption will never end. This change also must happen at the university level as I have described in detail on the simplistic and complex issues we are addressing.

Administration is currently notorious for having all the people who never were great teachers in the classroom or who just want to make more money. These individuals like to sit on the fence and shout that it is in the best interest of the children, but they really just teeter on the fence and fall on the side that will allow them to keep their job. "It requires a very unusual mind to make an analysis of the obvious" "If fifty million people say a foolish thing, it is still a foolish thing" (Kubik 1996).

Many administrators really drive little positive things in school. They often try to confine themselves to an echo chamber where the small group of people (usually other administrators, school board members, and possibly some teachers) can commiserate and mindlessly follow deficient government mandates without ever actually looking themselves in the mirror and realizing they are some of the most unimportant and irrelevant people in just about every aspect of life! They are particularly unimportant and irrelevant to the very students that they supposedly serve/help.

The most amazing thing I witnessed in my last years was the individual who somehow landed the director of curriculum position. I have always laughed at this because this individual was the ineptest leader as well as being the ineptest person with respect to curriculum itself. This person's role is to also provide professional development for teachers, which is even more embarrassing. What we end up getting is an individual who is making ninety to one hundred thousand dollars and becomes the biggest waste of time for teachers, has no leadership, and walks around with no clue. This scenario only happens in corrupt systems like schools where incompetent people keep getting paid and protected. If the individual had to enter the private sector where they are at the mercy of actually demonstrating that they have something valuable to teach, sell, and positively affect people, they would not have a job or any self-worth. This example is perfect to describe administration in the big picture.

Systems are always believing that their titles are more important than their actual abilities and knowledge/intelligence. Status quo is not excellence, and following government script is not leading or making important change. Remember, if fifty million people say something that is foolish, it is still foolish! Great spirits have always found violent opposition from mediocrities!

A final corrupt aspect to this problem is the teacher preparation programs at universities and colleges. There is a big disconnect between university teaching preparation programs and the actual ability it takes to be a great teacher. I have seen some colleges not having their physical education students even have contact with the exercise physiology teachers. How that is even remotely possible is very concerning to the ability to educate. When colleges drive the cardiovascular doctrine, technology in exercise that is driven by money and the status quo of "follow the science," then fitness and physical education will be set back to 1965 all over again. This follows the statement Verkhoshanky made in 1997 when he stated a similar idea about the Russian periodization that many high-level scientists tried to copy and pass off as the next magic bullet. The politics involved linking the colleges to public schools and collaborating to create curriculum makes it a difficult obstacle for needed curriculum changes in the teacher preparation programs, which then can begin to help the public school classroom.

Building relationships with the kids in my strength and conditioning program became the norm. One of the things I was highly recognized for, besides my physical education ideas, was the weight room program I developed in Pennsylvania. I had moved back from attending graduate school at Boise State University.

Boise State was a turning point in my life. I was working as an assistant under Joe Kenn and teaching on the floor, which was a tremendous experience. One day, I received a call around 5:30 in the morning and heard my mother's voice. I immediately knew that this was not good. She just quietly said that "your dad didn't make it." This was the worst day of my life to this point. Long story short is that I made a decision that I didn't really like the lifestyle of major college coaching. I did not like the constant moving every couple of years to get to where you thought you wanted to go. I did not like the politics where if you were doing a great job and being recognized as a great strength coach and the head football coach was fired, then your job was not safe because the new football coach was going to bring in their own person for your position. Never is this more evident than right now in the era of name image and likeness (NIL).

Everybody moves for money. It is more of a cult and who do you know. Some are very good, and some are just thought of as good more because who endorses them rather than it actually being a fact that the coach is good. With all the nonsense in education and sport with the money and self-serving agendas of television and universities and the fitness industry, I am extremely proud that two of the most important people in my life came from the University of Arkansas. Coach Stucky and Coach Campbell (Coach Campbell is a football coaching legend who coached under Bear Bryant at Alabama, was a very successful defensive coordinator at Oklahoma state, coached in the NFL, and, most importantly, coached me) are people who provided the example that much of our society has forgotten. Both are legends in their own right. Coach Stucky was a pioneer in strength and conditioning, and Coach Campbell takes a back seat to no one when it comes to coaching football at the division I level as well as his time in the NFL. Outside of all the accolades both men possess, the real hidden greatness is that both individuals were and are the best people you could choose to be around.

When I decided to move back to Pennsylvania and make a career out of teaching and coaching, I decided not to live in my hometown of Warren, Pennsylvania. I landed forty-two minutes away in rural Pennsylvania school. This was where all my experience and ideas poured out. The high school had no semblance of a weight room. They had a small L-shaped room with a squat rack and three benches and an incline rack. They had some dumbbells, and that was about it. I immediately started a strength and conditioning program and channeled my innermost Coach Stucky. I had little to work with, but we were going to bench, squat, and learn the classic weight lifts. I started with five football players and started adding a few girls in the first six months. The room was too small, so I had the weightlifting exercises out in the hallway. Only one football player could actually squat 315 pounds. As summer rolled around, word was getting out, and more kids started to want to lift. In less than a year, the number had grown to thirty or forty people.

As the beginning of the second lifting year came, we had at least fifteen kids squatting 315 pounds, and the rest is history. I developed the year-round strength and conditioning program, and I had kids from all sports (both girls and boys) as well as students who just wanted to learn to lift.

The administration was so pleased that they knocked out the wall between the little weight room and the wrestling room. I was given the forty by forty wrestling room and the existing little L-shaped room because of the success of my program. In a short time, I had fourteen squat racks and over one hundred lifters in the year-round strength and conditioning program. This would be ten percent of the student population at that time. I also built and funded the weight room without any grant money. We did it old school, and that is something I am very proud of!

Over the fifteen years of teaching at the high school level, I would be rich if I had a nickel for every time a student told me they would not have come to school if it weren't for the strength and conditioning program. Kids would show up at 6:00 a.m. just to hang out even though they lifted after school. Building relationships and developing a sense of pride in kids to desire to achieve is really what education should be about. The strength and conditioning program demonstrated that fact, and it was indisputable.

The strength and conditioning program also was a huge part of the physical education program as well, which is exactly the way it should be. This also created a great opportunity for the high school physical education program. You cannot have great physical education without the knowledge of great strength and conditioning. Both of those knowledge bases should go hand in hand. Ironically, ninety-nine percent of the colleagues I have been aware of have little to no knowledge of great strength and conditioning, and they all have been schooled in the cardiovascular doctrine, which means that great physical education cannot occur because of the status quo of information/education.

As previously described in the book, with cites from Siff, Verkhoshansky, Brehm, Tindell, Hackenschmidt, and Kubik, I am confident that very few graduating from colleges and becoming physical educators have had any knowledge of this information nor have they had any clue how to implement this knowledge to create a great physical education program.

To piggyback on the lack of knowledge, I want to enlighten you on a very true story of how deep the politics and corruption goes with the physical education echo chamber and self-promoters. I had had enough of the ridiculous claims of PE4life and the dog and pony shows that had been riding on my wife and I's knowledge to promote themselves. A lone colleague of mine at the time agreed with me, and she was willing to speak with me at the Pennsylvania state AAHPERD physical education conference. I never really wasted my time with these groups. I always wrote and drove my own curriculum with my knowledge and expertise for the kids. I never wanted to be affiliated with the corrupt trash that these echo chambers created. They were full of arrogance and ignorance as well. We had to turn in written forms for the title of our presentation, topics of information, etc.

Shortly after, PSEA AAHPERD called our department head at the time and felt that our presentation was negative towards the PE4life physical education agenda. I could not believe that a so-called educational entity that lays claim to pushing a positive agenda for physical education and kids would be so frightened at the thought that our presentation would not follow the bullshit they were pedaling. We had to have a classic corrupt meeting with an indoctrinated assistant superintendent. By the time I was done verifying the lies and corrupt practices of the department head, the assistant superintendent quickly supported what we were planning on presenting. This is a prime example of self-promoters creating an echo chamber of ignorance that does not like to be challenged. This is where the titles in the systems think they are important rather than actually having expertise or knowledge. Welcome to the dirty corruption, politics, and the uneducated educators who are teaching our children. The state AAHPERD group then got back to us and said they would like us to present. My colleague and I said absolutely not, and I moved on.

Name, image, and likeness (NIL) is currently the new movement. As stated previously, the shift now creates a college education system that is more tied to the professional sports echo chamber, money/television, and social media bonanza where every person wants their fifteen minutes of fame, hoping for their own perceived importance and wealth. This is a far cry from the year 1992. At that time, I was still a walk-on football player at the University of Arkansas, and I also was having the time of my life.

I remember a group of us players were sitting outside on a late Saturday evening. The group consisted of players who were likely going to make it to the NFL and the rest of us. We all were commenting that all players, even the walk-ons who help make a great team, should be getting money so we can have the luxury to eat out during the week. The amount of money the universities get from a major sport like football was growing larger by the day and fully funding other sports that allowed all of those sports to exist (especially due to Title IX). The argument, of course, back then was that the scholarship players already did not have to pay for school. Clearly, that thinking didn't realize that the issue was far more complex, and the money that we were talking about was simple things like going out to McDonalds or Taco Bell and having change for doing laundry. The new society with NIL is giving millions! That is a far cry from McDonalds and Taco Bell (ha ha)!

Television was beginning to nationalize games where previously it was regional exposure. I was fortunate enough to witness firsthand a legendary football program like Arkansas making the move to the SEC. I don't think many could foresee how big this move would become. I am sure that this move is the catalyst for what we now see today. Superconferences, the haves and have nots, little loyalty because in the end, everybody seems to want theirs, and money is the biggest part of it. There is a sports documentary about how Arkansas left the Southwest Conference for the SEC, and the upheaval it caused. Our head coach at the time stated that he was never told about the move and was never in the meetings. This speaks volumes to what we see in today's sports. This all was a great learning experience for me because as crazy as this world has become, there isn't a person in the world that can piss in the wind and tell me that it is raining!

A second big educational experience at the University of Arkansas occurred in 1991. We had a difficult task to open the season against the University of Miami (recognized as the U). The Hurricanes were very good and had been the premier college football program for the last decade at that time. As we were preparing to play this great team, the coaches had preached about the fact that the Hurricanes were so deep talent-wise that that was the mark of just how good they were. We understood that if you made a college team of the second, third, and fourth string players at the University of Miami, that team would actually be a top twenty team in its own right. The University of Miami at that time was exactly that.

The irony today is that you really won't see this in our current society likely ever again. This statement is definitely true and also formed a great piece of my philosophy in coaching and teaching in public schools. We should be creating a system of pride, loyalty, success, and intrinsic drive to succeed and excel! Also any great coach should develop every player, not just the most talented players. Through experience, the kids who are the best in junior high are not always the best by the time they become juniors in high school.

Speaking to football specifically, I do not want three good players and the rest just participating. I want a minimum of twenty-two good players with the other thirteen working and developing as well so we have thirty-five great players. Your last name doesn't matter, and playing time is earned, and all players work like division I players so they can reach a potential that they did not know they possessed. Remember, we do not try to reach our potential because none of us know what potential we actually have until we work appropriately to discover what that potential actually becomes. This idea should also be applied to a great physical education program. Coach Stucky's program did just that for me, and I passed that legendary knowledge on as well as advanced it.

Coaching and Public Schools

We now have things like NIL, transfer portal, and coaches leaving for big money almost exclusively under secrecy until the news can drop it on the public and create constant drama. Players do not care what jersey they put on, they just want to be paid and to have notoriety. Universities do not care if a great player comes for a year or two and then leaves because it's about winning and money. High school players are getting paid, and they have not even taken a snap in major college football yet. I remember Terry Bradshaw on an NFL pregame show about ten years ago saying that the NFL should not be paying these huge contracts to draft picks who have not even proven they can play at a high level for even one season. Bradshaw was one hundred percent correct. The ignorance and arrogance from the NFL has now reached even beyond the major college ranks. Now high school players are getting the money and deals, and those players too have not played a snap for a major college program. I see kids on YouTube promoting themselves when they are not even close to being as good as they think they are, yet this is how things are, and it will have to implode for society to rein in all of what has been created presently. "ESPN published a report by Dan Murphy about the academic bonus payments (up to $5980 per year), allowed by the U.S. Supreme Court's decision in the NCAA v. Alston money. Nick Saban addressed the matter in the opening statement of his Wednesday press conference, 'The Alston money, we pay our players that,' Saban said. 'We paid them last semester, we're paying them this semester'" (Olson 2022). The Alston case allows schools to pay academic bonuses.

ESPN senior writer Chris Low also reported an interview of Clemson head football coach, Dabo Swinney. Swinney, in my opinion, has given the best national response to this entire mess. He also is the only high-level person I have heard at this time to come out and speak real truth to what we have addressed in this book on these issues. Swinney stated, "I think there's going to be a complete blowup…especially in football, and there needs to be." Swinney said the current system is a mess, and that its's hard to get anything accomplished as college athletics continue to evolve and change in the new world of the transfer portal and NIL. "There's so much bureaucracy, and you can't get anything done in a real-time manner. It's frustrating. The communication is not good, and the rules are outdated." This statement is exactly what we have been documenting and outlining with exercise, public schools, and the many problems that have led us to why physical education has been destroyed.

In the school district that I have been referring to, any students who participate in a sport do not need to have physical education, the students are exempt. I have observed that many kids do just that in sports in many schools. They just participate! Many are out of shape, many are not even remotely good at the sport, and they are not physically fit by any means. Yet they do not need to take physical education. Clearly, the very people who claim to be educated demonstrate they are the furthest thing from being educated. In fact, they are the complete antithesis and are very ignorant. This is a prime example why we felt it a necessity to write this book and try to get great physical education recognized.

Swinney went on to say, "There's no rules, no guidance, no nothing." Swinney said "It's out of control. It's not sustainable. It's an absolute mess and a train wreck, and the kids are going to be the ones who suffer in the end. There are going to be a lot of kids that end up with no degrees and make decisions based on the wrong things" (Low, 2022). These statements by Coach Swinney encompass everything we have written in this book! The plight of physical education is exactly due to the mess and train wreck from many complex networks. We set out to describe our professional experience and expertise to address every aspect so education (specifically physical education) can return and take its rightful prominence and importance in all people's lives!

All that we have just discussed has created another alarming status quo in youth sports through high school. The quest to be seen by a college coach has become fanatical. Youth sports grades 3–6 are running travel leagues with often a mom or dad coaching the sport with little to no experience. The biggest understanding that many of these coaches have is that they watch the sport on television and then try to have the eight-year-olds emulate the play or training program they watched on TV or YouTube. Sport specialization has been around for a long time, but the new society we have been speaking of has taken it to all towns in the country. Just in the small town I live in, we have a low population, and we have every sport trying to specialize year-round. The talent level is minimal, so the brilliant people then create AAU and travel teams both out of town and within the tiny town.

Now we have kids playing on three different basketball or soccer teams, and some or all the coaches threaten the kids that if they play for the other team and miss practice, then they will lose playing time for his/her team even though the kids I am speaking about are the best players. We play youth tackle football, and kids sit the bench in third grade with the quest of winning even though six years later, none of the players are even remotely good at football at the high school level. Not letting third graders play because they are not good makes no sense when the league is supposed to be developing these young players who have an interest or love for football. You would think the light bulb would come on that putting helmets and shoulder pads on third graders likely will not result in being a great football player later on. This example has been going on for over twenty years, and the level of football players only gets worse, and yet the school system and adults have no clue. "It requires a very unusual mind to make an analysis of the obvious" (Alred North Whitehead). It should be easy to see where this is going.

To add to this entirely ridiculous situation, it is the high school sports running full games in the off-season and competing with the club teams. All these are occurring in a school system that only graduates 125 kids per class if they are lucky. It is easy to see that this leads to kids burning out, quitting, and not actually learning to work so they can get better during their young life. Winners do things that losers do not want to do, so now the losers underperform and are told how good they are. All this giant lie then creates the next lazy and crazy set of parents, and the cycle becomes the same rehash of the old trash, and nothing seems to change. All sport factions are split, and all are trying to load their team in the name of winning, and trust me, no kids are winning in this situation.

The school I am referring to also had three suicides within weeks. This had never happened before and especially in such a small quiet town. Mental health is currently the new crisis added to this ever-changing landscape. Exercise alone has been proven to help with this, and the training I am speaking about is vastly better than the exercise promoted and sold under the cardiovascular doctrine. It is very clear that the schools are struggling with the mental health of their students and much of it can be linked to the ridiculous state testing and the behavior in school from the woke and cancel cultures that are inundating the schools. The kids are completely overwhelmed, and the bureaucracy that is public education cannot cut through the politics to actually change even though that is exactly their motto. Every administrator who speaks has been talking about how change is occurring, but they really miss the point. The change is not in increasing testing. The change is not just simply adding technology and still running the same structured environment as the 1920s. The change is not eliminating the arts and physical education for more rigor.

Realistically, everything about public schools needs to change. A specific change that needs to happen is one that is demonstrated in other countries successfully and yet the United States ignores. In Finland, their focus is on daily physical activity and happiness and literally none of the rest of what the US education system attempts to do (e.g., vast amounts of testing). Finland mandates one hour of recess and physical activity every day. Their children are happy and learn social skills. The United States still cannot figure out why we deal with so many school shootings, and yet it is clear that the bureaucracy has taken complete control of the United States public education system, and its policy and practices are at the heart of all the problems. Public education will continue spewing its corrupt words and policies and shout that they are for change, but it really is not changing and continues to chase its tail spiraling downward on a daily basis.

Remember the quotes from Albert Einstein and T. S. Elliot. "Great spirits have always found violent opposition from mediocrities!" Elliot stated, "Humankind cannot bear very much reality!" These two quotes sum up the political corruption we have been speaking about. The reality is that physical education that does not follow the cardiovascular doctrine is likely the most important class children can take. Mental health and happiness are more important than the fake rigor of government-driven curriculum and completely ridiculous state testing exams that absolutely do not indicate that a person is more intelligent.

To add to this warped reality, the school system itself chooses to not do anything to remedy the situation with these poor coaching examples sometimes because the school knows there is nobody else to fill the position. That is not a position that force 46 can support. School policy and the athletic directors should be at the forefront to halt the specialization and poor coaching within the community, and if the ADs can't deal with the situation, then like most things in life, the AD needs to find another career, and the school needs to hire a new AD. It is an easy fix though. I spoke on how to train the multisport athlete most of my career with the NSCA and as state director. The key is strength and conditioning year-round and well developed, vertically aligned great physical education programs, not playing sports year-round. This may sound too simplistic, but it is just that. Understanding strength and conditioning would eliminate all this nonsense because what happens is the kids who are in my strength and conditioning program outshine by a landslide the kids who haphazardly train and try and play six sports.

Secondary to this is removing the status quo administrators and school board members when they are ignoring serious problems. As public school educators in the state of Pennsylvania, we are required to prove that we do not have a history of abusing children. We must submit clearances from the FBI that prove that we have not and do not participate in criminal activity. We are required by Pennsylvania State mandate to report any suspicion or knowledge of physical/emotional abuse of the kids we are bound to protect. Yet many of these very same kids are at the mercy of coaches who don't seem to care for their safety. Inappropriate overtraining of sports participants, poorly run and specialized year-round sports programs that require athletes to choose between one coach's practices and those of other coaches', and threatening playing time (e.g., often one in-season sport versus one out-of-season sport going on at the same time) are plainly and simply abuse! This abuse is both physical and emotional by nature.

When you see sport coaches at the youth through high school level trying to run practices all year long and threatening kids with losing playing time because they do not attend their ridiculous practices and nothing gets done about it, then there should be real concern and consequences for these coaches and school districts. When a soccer coach somehow thinks his/her expertise is strength and conditioning for the sport that they coach, then there should be real concern and consequences for these coaches and school that sit and do nothing. Running eighth grade girls five miles multiple times per week to get in condition is so ridiculous and outdated that you would think these coaches are living in 1975.

This particular soccer coach actually made a statement to the girls that you have to squat two hundred pounds and bench one hundred pounds to play. The public school officials statement is that the coach can run their program as they see fit! The reality check needs to be that being a sport coach does not mean that you are a strength coach. A soccer coach whose professional job is being a photographer with no real accolades in playing or coaching soccer should not then be trying to hold ridiculous workouts that do nothing but overtrain kids and most certainly do not help the kids reach the unknown potential that they have. This particular soccer coach actually told the girls that a soccer player typically runs seven miles in a game, so running multiple days of five miles in the summer will somehow make the kids great soccer players. Apparently, this brilliant photographer claiming to be a soccer coach has not seen the VO_2 max study cited earlier in the book. Then the coach adds to the stupidity by running strength and conditioning periods, having no knowledge on what strength and conditioning is. Running five miles then doing planks then doing medicine ball tosses for ninth grade soccer girls is an absolute joke of a training concept! Ironically, the girls who have been running five miles for two months get very fatigued just doing five reps on a squat clean. This is a clear example of why running five miles becomes outdated and irrelevant for literally all sports and why wannabe coaches need to not coach!

Another example to piggyback off the running five miles to get in shape would be the fact that I had the great fortune of training an outstanding individual to prepare to go to West Point out of high school. I had been training Ben Amsler for three or four years, and he became a poster child for what great training and effort every day should look like. Toward the end of his senior year, he stated he wanted to get ready for heading to West Point. Simply, we did not need to change too much, and I specifically told him he really did not need to run more than one time per week. I had an emphasis day for specific conditioning in the weight room, and his testimonial on my website says it all. Ben graduated commander of the corp (highest ranking cadet) at West Point, and I proudly watched him lead Army out for the Army-Navy game.

As a fourteen year old kid, I pushed back on Coach T in weight room knowledge believing my men's fitness magazine education knew better, yet I listened to Coach and I got stronger. By age eighteen, I listened to every word coach had to say and by the time I left high school for The United States Military Academy, I was pound for pound the strongest I have ever been to this point. I excelled in basic training because of the strength I built in Coach's weight room. Coach enforced perfect techniques, and once you mastered movements, he pushed you to the limit (often redefining what I thought were limits). Through the years of playing sports, four years at West Point, five years in the Army with two combat tours and now ultra-running, I have yet to experience a serious injury. I attribute this to Coach's balanced approach and relentless focus on total body strength. I have taken and used Coach T's methods throughout my life. Though I was never as strong as the day I walked out of his weight room, I took what I learned and applied it to my nine years in uniform. At West Point and in the Army, you are required to complete a PT test twice per year. The test consists of two minutes of push-ups, two minutes of sit ups, and a 2-mile run. As a result, people in uniform spend a lot of time doing these three exercises. Many of these officers and soldiers were very good at the PT test but faltered and failed when they were required to actually execute the tasks required of them in training and combat. I witnessed top scoring soldiers unable to continue their mission in the heat of battle because of a lack of strength. When I entered West Point, I continued to use what I learned from Coach and never focused on the bi-yearly PT tests until two weeks prior to ensure my form and technique was correct. I received a top score in every PT test I executed in school and in the army while also being able to lead soldiers through every situation imaginable. The Army is just now starting to catch up to where Coach T was twenty years ago with new requirements for testing soldiers. The Army and its soldiers will need to learn what Coach has been teaching since the beginning, they will need to learn how to grow and maintain true strength. Coach T's programs and approach to strength are always evolving. His methods have been and continue to be twenty years ahead of his peers and the general public. Whether you are an athlete, in the military, interested in service in a physically demanding profession, or just a person that wants to lose weight, Coach T can help get you there. I am thankful that I learned my lesson twenty years ago. Listen to Coach T and your body will exceed any expectations that you set for it! (Amsler)

The specifics on my role in helping Ben could be for another book, but the point is that he lifted free weights the John Stucky and force 46 way, and he used no machines, and we placed no effort on running miles and miles multiple times a week. Even ultramarathon athletes can be trained most of their annual plan in the weight room without running if they are around a strength and conditioning coach who knows what they are actually doing. Of course, the standard ignorance of these coaches always use the latest buzzwords like "We are going to train our core," "We are going to functionally train," or "We are going to engage in sport specific training" (LOL… soccer players typically run seven miles in a game, so let's have thirteen-year-old girls run five miles three times per week so they can get in shape).

We also see the basketball coach bring in a certified trainer from the YMCA, and this clown actually takes all basketball players and has them jump off stacked forty-five-pound plates, holding a medicine ball, attempting to do a high-level plyometrics with kids who have not developed the strength to even deal with their body weight let alone try to be explosive with a weight.

As stated earlier, the strength and conditioning I am speaking about is exactly what drives a great physical education program. I already have demonstrated this fact over my twenty-five years, so that is all that needs to be said. The root of all this knowledge is what I specifically learned from Coach Stucky, and the rest is history! This is exactly why this book had to be written. This book is about learning from the best, continually growing and improving knowledge, personally training and coaching many thousands of kids from Kindergarten through the division I level over the last twenty-five years that I cannot even guess the actual number of human beings I actually have trained. Also this is not just about people going to play in college, it is about actual long-term lifetime fitness and how physical education can teach this to all kids to take care of themselves for the rest of their life whether it is the nonathlete or the athlete who is done playing and needs to maintain great fitness or the aspiring athlete who has an opportunity to play in college.

The reality of addressing a great training program becomes even more complex when you add the media and current trends of competition that has been promoted with bodybuilding, CrossFit competition, and thousands of one-thousand-pound dead lifts and back squats on Google News, YouTube, and Twitter. No Division 1 strength coach gave CrossFit any credence when it first was marketed. Currently, of course, CrossFit has become a competition that now creates a new proprietary program packaged as training properly, which then trickles down to the high schools and middle schools and gym classes and becomes the next false narrative of really good training. This also leads these future parents to become just as ignorant as the cardiovascular doctrine believers and wannabe sport coaches who were lucky to have even played well at the JV level during their high school years.

Marcus Filly spoke a very real truth in a recent article. Marcus was a former CrossFit games contender. He has figured out what any of the true strength coaches understand. CrossFit is all about taking high-level appropriate lifts (if taught by a true strength and conditioning coach) and paying little attention to reps, sets, volume, and rest.

> MARCUS FILLY DOESN'T want you pounding out rounds of EMOM (i.e. every minute on the minute) thrusters until your shoulders can barely move, and he doesn't want you going so hard during Murph that you're a quivering mess when you finally finish. Yes, the former CrossFit Games contender knows pile-driving past fatigue is a CrossFit staple, and he understands why you think the secret to building muscle and strength is always to just work harder. But the veteran coach has other ideas. And Filly has seen what

that leads to: It may blast calories and help you build muscle in the short term, but it can lead to diminishing results over the long haul. It usually causes burnout. From running to bodybuilding, too much of the fitness industry pushes you to chase fatigue above all else. "Blow through all your mental, emotional, and physical resources in your workouts and you're not going to have the same capacity for your job, wife, husband, or other interests," says Filly. You're seeking better health, but you're actually robbing yourself of it, he says. (Heffernan 2022)

I recently saw a news article where a fitness app actually promoted three lifting choices for programs. You are able to click on a program for "getting shredded," you are able to click on a program for building strength, and you are able to click on a program for losing weight. My clients and I get a real laugh at the new fitness movement because we get all these things from our training philosophy that is promoting great training the way the human body should be trained. Coach Stucky was doing this many years ago, and force 46 is just the extension of the template of what he taught.

The New PE

In 2019, the CDC stated only 7 percent of kids worldwide meet the recommended activity threshold every week. In the United States, this problem is magnified! In 2016, a *British Journal of Medicine* study demonstrated that America's youth ranked forty-seventh out of fifty countries who had their activity level measured. Jim Baugh, founder of PHIT America, believes that America's dilemma can be defeated through a revival of local physical education programs (www.phitamerica.org). We believe this is true, however, the corruption, proprietary programming, self-promotion, and school political culture has always stood in the way of great physical education to solve this problem.

This book is intended to set the standard of great physical education that overcomes all the obstacles that my wife and I have battled through to answer the questions. We have demonstrated this for our individual classes, but the message has to get out to the entire United States and then the results will be readily observed.

Baugh traces the roots of inactivity to two important factors: "kids today no longer are able to develop the skills to become lifelong athletes and this absence of requisite skills results in a lack of confidence needed to pursue activity." Ironically, this is the exact theme the new PE and PE4life packaged and sold to school districts and the United States population at large. Also this idea was driven by the insurance companies, the cardiovascular doctrine, and, of course, the money-driven machine weight companies with enormous amounts of money at stake. Force 46 physical education understands that the new PE and physical educators need to stop inventing comparisons and labeling athletes versus Nonathletes.

Siff 2003 states, "The essence of sport is human movement." The fact is that physical educators need to develop human movement in vertical alignment from Pre-K through grade 12 and stop the nonsense of making statements that gym class should not be for the athletes. Every person needs to develop the movement abilities whether they choose to be an athlete or a nonathlete. All the physical education movements from 1965 to current time have not addressed this in a correct or complete sequence, which is a huge problem.

One of the best books written on movement, in our opinion, is *Movement with a Purpose: Perceptual Motor-Lesson Plans for Young Children*. This book that was published in 1983 and written by Madeleine Brehm and Nancy T. Tindell was very much correct, and for whatever reason, physical education did not follow their lead, and things only became worse to current times. A large portion of our students are deficient in most, if not all, areas of the S-factors that Siff and Verkohshansky cited. Most physical educators that we have come across in our almost sixty years of experience do not recognize what fitness actually is or how it is displayed. The only opportunity for many of our kids to engage in play and appropriate/necessary movement is in their physical education class, and as society keeps changing, things will likely only get worse.

The brain-muscle link that is so inherent in weightlifting is also inherent in great physical education design. Siff 2003 states the following with respect to the brain-muscle link:

> Cognitive plyometrics is the preparatory period prior to the plyometric action that can involve higher-order mental processing of exceptional intricacy (running mental pictures). The brain plays a central role in orchestrating muscular movement (not solely neuromuscular) (Evarts, n.d.). Even though the same muscles may be involved in a movement, they may be controlled by different parts of the brain depending on the speed of movement. (Siff 2003)

> When observing the heart circulatory system, isometric and dynamic exercise recruit different brain mechanisms due to increase in blood pressure but little increase in blood flow. Dynamic exercise, on the other hand, generates an O^2 demand that is largely met by increase in the volume of blood pumped and a decrease resistance to its flow. To complicate matters further, slow as opposed to rapid execution of the same movement might involve different muscle groups. This is muscles alive! (Siff 2003)

> When addressing the mind issue, it is observable that the average fitness devotee wants quick fixes that require little additional work or single-minded concentration. (Siff 2003)

This can be attributed to the cardiovascular doctrine itself. "How strongly does the mind become involved in any gym exercise if you use light unchallenging movements, loads, reps, sets, and workouts" (Siff 2003)?

This should sound familiar because this is exactly the cardiovascular doctrine. "Under these conditions, the mind can go on holiday, keep almost entirely out of the training process, and even allow you to read, talk, or watch television while you are exercising" (Siff 2003). This belief system has brought fitness, exercise, and physical education in the United States to the point we are currently at.

> Let's look at the opposite scenario. Use heavyweights, high-intensity methods, heavy super-slow, near maximal loads, reps, reps to failure or novel training variations (like our barrels), concentration curls, minimal rest intervals, and other very demanding or challenging training strategies. Under these conditions, there is no chance to let the mind relax, take a hike elsewhere, watch television, and complete the exercise effectively! (Siff 2003)

Quality physical education should not have fluff, political interference, or incompetent proprietary programming where there is a trail of self-promotion and money! The brain-muscle link is extremely important to the ability of children to learn as well. This is why we developed high-level academic interventions through physical education class.

Movement with a Purpose: Perceptual Motor-Lesson Plans for Young Children (Brehm and Tindell 1983) again speaks to things my wife and I both developed to a high level in our schools pertaining to academic learning. The academic attributes of *Movement with a Purpose: Perceptual Motor-Lesson Plans for Young Children* state that it is a well-known fact that children learn and remember most when actively and physically involved in a learning situation. Eye/hand coordination gained through motor skills can have a bearing on the manner in which a child writes to express all that intellectual potential. Seriation, the ability to recreate movements in a series, has its counterpart in academic tasks such as spelling and reading. Being judged as a success in games witnessed and valued by peers will help any child's self-esteem to grow, and that child may try harder in the intellectual realm. This last point has totally been destroyed since 1983 with the noncompetitive movement, everybody gets a trophy cult, the societal soccer mom mentality and the no one loses mob!

(Not very) recently in the physical education world, there began a push to minimize sports and competition from the PE setting and replace it with packaged programs and activities that focused instead on self-exploration, challenge by choice, and so-called lifetime skills. They are calling it the new PE. Every time we turn around, there is a new article or new study or a new program promoting this much improved concept of the new PE. I began with "(not very) recently" because there is really nothing new about this concept at all. It's been going on for years. Some schools just seem to be a little behind in jumping on the bandwagon. The problem with this new PE concept is that it just might not be *great* PE at all!

The new PE promotes fitness on treadmills and expensive machines that typically require grant funding. The new PE promotes the use of pedometers and no-team sports. The new PE promotes challenge by choice, rock wall, and FitGram testing along with lifetime sports. If this sounds familiar, it should. This is very similar to Western Periodization, plyometrics, aerobic exercise. "Lifting weights makes you big," "lifting weights makes you slow," "lifting weights is bad for your knees," "whole grain is good for you" (oh wait, wheat is now genetically modified), the Atkins diet, walking ten thousand steps a day is healthy and fun, etc.

The new PE, along with many university physical education teacher programs, pushed the narrative that dodgeball has to be eliminated because it encouraged strong people to pick on weak people or athletes versus nonathletes.

Some questions I have been asking are, Dodgeball is somehow inappropriate in our current times of student depressions, anxiety / testing burnout, and school shootings?

In all my years of teaching jail ball (a more active form of dodgeball), I have never seen this to be true. Also it is the teacher that sets the classroom management and expectations, so it is not the dodgeball game itself that is the problem! It is that the adult does not run the classroom correctly. The huge echo chamber that resulted from these kinds of statements caused the PE4life nonsense and poor teacher preparation programs at the universities. "It isn't that they can't see the solutions. It is that they can't see the problem" (G. K. Chesterton). T. S. Elliot stated, "Humankind cannot bear very much reality."

Great PE recognizes that our kids need to move, and they need to gain control of their bodies. Whether this is done using sports skills and implements or the treadmill and pedometers is where new PE and great PE differ. One area of learning where new PE falls short is the lack of emphasis on *play* and a corresponding push on *programs*. Plain and simple, kids need to play. If it is not enjoyable, it is not likely to be repeated. Not only do kids benefit from the physical movement of play, but they also learn social and safety skills that do not present themselves while pedaling on a stationary bike. Research has shown that play is important to healthy development of the brain. Free play (more child-driven) promotes creative problem solving and the development of leadership and group skills. Structured play (adult-driven) encourages fairness, sharing, and resiliency. It gives students the opportunity to practice self-regulation and decision-making skills.

The new PE has allowed lazy teachers who cannot develop a true fun environment for kids that demands high expectations of great effort, teamwork, fun, owning their own behavior, and respect. The new PE likes to complain that so many PE teachers just rolled out the ball and played games. Like any profession, I am sure there are a percentage of PE teachers who did that just like the many doctors and lawyers are guilty of malpractice, school board members who are corrupt, administrators who do nothing and collect a bigger paycheck than the very professionals who actually are helping the kids, or the corrupt priest in the Catholic church, or the corrupt police officer, and yes, even the corrupt practices of many members of congress…I hope you get the point.

Great PE is driven by play and willful participation. It is reinforced by practice and repetition of crucial movement skills and patterns. It teaches our students the benefits of exercise and how to maintain a suitable level for wellness and fitness. It is *not* driven by skills tests, expensive machines, or proprietary programs. Early movement skill development is one of the single greatest short falls in today's PE classes. Again the fitness craze that was prevalent in the early 1980s—which now is packaged as fitness machines, heart rate monitors, and pedometers—do not develop movement skills. Also the concept of actual play, which we have stated, is far more important than the fitness push that so many experts and self-promoting followers of the new PE are advocating.

Let's take a look at the lifetime activities versus team sports stance. It simply should not even be an issue. Sports are sports! Any sport requires skills. Whether it is one we can continue to enjoy individually and into our old age or limited to the young and strong, sports require the same skills we need in lifetime movement and fitness. It's not about sports at all. It's about teaching our kids how to take care of their bodies, how to be prepared for vigorous activity, and how to maintain a level of strength, respiratory fitness, and flexibility that leads to comfort and ease of movement in later years. Teaching "team sports" in physical education does not mean we foster competition, intimidation, frustration, or exclusion. Team sports require important movement skills that can be very effectively practiced in small group/noncompetitive settings. Just because a teacher teaches the skill of basketball shooting, dribbling, passing, or dodging, does not designate the class as "team sports" based. It should, most appropriately, be movement based.

You need to look at the benefits of types of movements and manipulations to determine if they have a place in a PE program. Take dribbling, for example, one might argue the significance of dribbling practice to a student who may never intend to participate in a basketball game. But if you look at the actual skill of dribbling, you will see far more than a means of advancing on a court without carrying the ball! It involves eye-hand coordination (necessary for the development of writing, shoe tying, zipping a coat, catching a tossed item). It requires visual motor control, tracking, beat competency, fine motor control, and large motor control—all extremely relevant skills in cognitive development and learning as well as physical education. Fitness has married itself with not "catering to athletes in PE class," yet striking, kicking, throwing, strength, flexibility, and movement mechanics are essential for elementary children and essential for a future of an active lifestyle. Unfortunately, after many years of teaching, I have yet to witness this going on in most PE classes. What I have seen is a lot of self-serving, self-promoting individuals wanting to push "improved PE programs" and using a poor teacher as the example for the masses.

This is also a good place to address the relationship between strength and gender. The book *Supertraining* cites many studies that have shown that the strength of a woman is approximately two-thirds of that of a male of the same body mass and age, with both male and female reaching peak strength at about the same age. This difference is largely due to the greater percentage of lean muscle mass in the male because muscle strength in males and females is virtually the same (four kilograms per square centimeter cross-sectional area).

> Studies (Hettinger 1961) have also revealed that there is a different strength ratio for different muscle groups in the male and female. These ratios are consistent with other research that reveals that upper body strength in women generally tends to be lower than that of men of equivalent body mass. They probably reflect the differences in type and intensity of work undertaken by the average man and woman in daily life, and it is likely that such differences will decrease or disappear among similarly trained male and female athletes. (Stiff 2003)

That is exactly true, and our society created the myths that women are weaker, girls can do push-ups on their knees, etc. The fact is that if girls/women were educated and inspired to actually train in the strength and conditioning realm as what my wife and I believe, then the myths and echo chambers that derived from the cardiovascular doctrine could be extinguished, and physical education programs could be a big piece in the quality of life for everyone!

The new PE loves to sell the FitGram testing program along with a computer program so you can pretest and posttest every child. That is really ironic because most elementary programs have PE only one day per week, which is a crime in and of itself. Why would you pretest and posttest a child when you only see them one day per week for nine months? And if you are running a great PE program, you certainly are not wasting their one day with running them on a treadmill or even running them outside because it won't be long before every child in your school will hate to run!

I taught for fifteen years in a nationally recognized high school PE program that utilized the FitGram testing program. One of the FitGram measures of fitness was a bicep curl test! Assessing the strength of an individual's bicep and then stating you are teaching kids how to be healthy is one of the most ignorant and embarrassing things I have ever witnessed. I also watched this as I was a two-term state director for the NSCA, and I felt things had to change. The unionized political system that is public education believes in following the status quo. Everybody's opinion is equal even if their résumés tell a different story. If a person does not follow the status quo, then you are not a team player. These mission statements from the schools and any big business system are nothing but corruption and living a complete lie. Things have not changed, but I believe, in many respects, they have become worse, so that is a big reason why those professionals who have done such great work in physical education can speak out against the politics and proprietary programming that has taken hold of our profession.

Getting back to FitGram testing in elementary PE, we shouldn't overlook the fact that you can't keep and promote this kind of data because the fitness benefits many students get are not solely tied to physical education class. For example, my son plays hockey three nights a week and then plays one to two games on the weekend every week from October to March, so the PE teacher who only sees him one day a week pretests his fitness in September and then in May. Do you really think his high fitness level is due to the one day per week PE class or do you think his high fitness level is due to his participation in hockey? Obviously, it is because of hockey as well as the other sports he plays. On top of that, the new PE will gather the data on kids like my son and then claim their PE program is showing great fitness benefits. The reality is it is important to teach and expose our kids to many things so they hopefully will make better choices on how to stay fit over their lifetime.

The one thing we know for sure is that aerobic exercise, treadmills, snowshoeing, and rock wall are not what kids will actually adhere to nor does this cover what fitness really is. Most students hate the fitness center and want to play games. If physical educators want to expose kids to outdoor education, there might be room in a day for it, but it should never be considered physical education. AAHPERD did the very same thing politically many years ago when it added the letter D at the end of their mission. The D stands for dance, and that was a political movement to include an echo chamber groups desire for their personal agenda to be advanced. There is nothing wrong with dance. It can be great exercise, but it is not something that should be forced upon children as a separate activity. Our children often dance in the strength agility skill stations out of happiness and joy, and that is not teacher-driven, and we feel that is the way it should be.

Twenty years ago, when heart rate monitors were becoming the next magic bullet in the new PE machine, I challenged the fitness center myth of fitness versus a basketball unit in the gym. Both the fitness center and all basketball players wore heart rate monitors. Both classes each had about twenty-five minutes of activity. Most of the people in the fitness center earned zeros or one point because they hated to be there, and the few that did want to actually work out in the fitness center earned about twenty-four minutes in the zone (140–180). At the end of the small group basketball games, most of my students recorded four to six minutes in the target heart rate. All the students recorded nineteen plus minutes over the zone, which means they worked above 180 BPM, playing like most people should learn to play. Very few, if any, of the basketball selection actually played on the basketball team as well. I did this study because I already understood that THR training is not all what it's cracked up to be, plus I wanted to demonstrate that the vast majority of students want to play games vigorously and cooperatively, and those classes will get far greater fitness benefits rather than being stuck on a stationary piece of equipment.

The new PE doesn't like team sports, but team sports are not the problem. It is all about how you develop the culture of your school! If everybody plays vigorously and safely, owns their own behavior, and plays with respect, then I will take small group team sports, along with human movement development anytime, over the fluff and proprietary programing of skateboarding, pedometers, cup stacking, snowshoeing, and treadmills! More importantly, so would all my students! But instead, the new PE would rather promote "challenge by choice." If the student chooses not to challenge himself, where is the growth and the learning? Would this be appropriate if Joey chooses to avoid subtraction problems during math because subtraction is new and unfamiliar? Or is this acceptable because he happens to be a wiz in addition? If we don't challenge our students, they will learn to avoid difficult situations—the very situations that foster high self-esteem, personal confidence, and pride in oneself. I have noticed that some individuals, specifically college professors who supervise student teachers, appear to be misinterpreting differentiated instruction with challenge by choice. It is our view that these two terms are very different. We do differentiate when appropriate, but many times, you can develop small-group lead up games with similar high expectations.

Brain-based learning is very much something that we do agree with in the new PE (except I think they drastically self-promote themselves for uncovering this piece of knowledge). However, what people really should understand is that all exercise has a benefit to learning whether it is dribbling a basketball, jogging, throwing a ball off the wall and catching it, or playing structured or unstructured games, and yes, that includes team sports! The elementary building I worked at, as well as my wife's K4–K5 building, were extremely supportive for our academic interventions through physical education concepts. The students played and exercised in the concepts presented throughout this book, and it had nothing to do with aerobic exercise or challenge by choice. The science is very clear and correct about the importance of daily physical education, yet our educational guru's, along with corrupt school board members with their own political self-interests, sit around a table monthly, scratching their heads as to why the test scores are getting worse as they continue to cut the arts time to sit our children in desks that create a poor learning environment where kids just do what they have to do to get out of the school. There is little new with respect to exercise and the brain. Many books and articles have been published, yet it seems as though I should list a couple in the book just in case a person has been asleep over the last thirty years or more.

> Exercise can turn your brain into a powerhouse of pleasure. Exercise stimulates a rich concoction of feel-good chemicals in the brain, including dopamine, serotonin, endocannabinoids, and norepinephrine. Not only do you produce more but your brain better enjoys them. According to the *Greater Good Science Center* (greatergood.berkeley.edu), exercise is so good at delivering pleasure to the brain that it's successfully used to help patients suffering from the ravaging aftereffects of drug abuse. It has been estimated that we all lose approximately thirteen percent of our dopamine receptors each decade, causing us to experience diminishing pleasure in everyday life as we age, and exercise can reverse this. (SciTechDaily)

Harvard Health Publishing (health.harvard. edu) reported that exercise sparks neurogenesis that is the formation of new neurons in the brain. We all are born with approximately one hundred billion neurons in the brain that regenerate at a fast rate in our childhoods but then slow as we mature. It was believed that this regeneration eventually stops completely. It has since been proven that neurogenesis can last a lifetime. (SciTechDaily)

The fact that exercise improves learning, and memory has been documented and written about in many articles and books. The book *Brain Rules* by Dr. Rattey was highly recognized. The only problem with the book was how it tried to advertise the old cardiovascular doctrine of Kenneth Cooper. Lifting weights does the same thing, but I would easily argue way better, so why chase your tail. Ironically, what do our public schools do instead? Our brilliant educational leaders get rid of physical education to make way for government-controlled accountability and knowledge to create a false sense of intelligence and academic rigor. As we have stated throughout this book, physical education is an absolute must on a daily basis for all kids, we just believe that this book is the correct guide.

"Exercise is one of the leading forms of therapy for people suffering from age-related dementia and Alzheimer," said the APA. It is a leading form of therapy because of its documented boost to memory function. Studies have shown that the hippocampus can increase in volume by one percent after a year of regular exercise. (SciTechDaily)

Our exercise program details our view of what the exercise should consist of. My wife and I have seen it all and have put together a clear picture of what physical education should be in a vertically aligned curriculum, and it's not expensive fitness centers with machines that require state and federal funding put into the hands of very confused physical educators and public school agents.

A profoundly classic status quo education hypothesis from known correct scientific information comes from a fourth benefit to improve brain function.

> Exercise can increase the thickness of the cerebral cortex. The cerebral cortex is associated with high-level conscious thought patterns that include emotion, evaluation, reasoning, and language. Johns Hopkins Medicine (hopkinsmedicine.org) stated that exercise can thicken the cerebral cortex. Researchers speculate that some of the reason for this is that exercise, particularly aerobic, involves continually making split-second decisions. If you are running, you are always managing your environment so you do not twist your ankle or tangle with a car. If you are working out in your gym, you are keeping your balance and monitoring your levels of exhaustion and thirst. In other words, your mind is working just as hard as your body. The result of this is a thicker, stronger cerebral cortex. (SciTechDaily)

We have already addressed the idea of researchers speculating that exercise, particularly aerobic, involves continually making split decisions in the earlier chapter dealing with mind-muscle link.

Researchers here still love to say aerobic for everything, and yet the clear evidence that Verkhoshansky and Siff cited from way back in the sixties and seventies shows that weightlifting is profoundly more enticing to the brain. You do not even need an expert to tell you this. Go out for a jog one day, and the next day, perform the clean and jerk or barbell snatch! Which exercise continually makes the cerebral cortex make split decisions? Lifting weights, like I program design in my business, will give you forty minutes to an hour of continual intense split decisions and cognitive thought that stationary equipment cannot even approach. This also speaks to why daily physical education for kids is so necessary in schools! People need to be an informed consumer when reading research and be able to read between the lines. I learned this in my graduate-level research and design class at Boise State University and again brings me right back to Coach Stucky! Coach has to be smiling at this book right now!

A *Washington Post* article titled "Exercise Boosts the Brain—and Mental Health," reported that new research reveals how physical activity can reduce and even ward off depression, anxiety, and other psychological ailments. Again this has been known for decades, yet the education system has deliberately chased the academic rigor nonsense and completely false narrative of intelligence by eliminating physical education and its importance.

> Mental health disorders such as depression and anxiety aren't easy to treat. Medications help many but have a high failure rate and may bring nasty side effects. Talk therapy is time-consuming and expensive. Neither approach is suited to preventing the disorders from developing in the first place. Many people overlook another option that, when it works, can be one of the most effective, least disruptive, and cheapest ways of managing mental health disorders: exercise. (Holmes 2022)

"It's hardly news that exercise is good for your physical health and has long been extolled as beneficial for mental health as well. But researchers are now making progress in understanding how exercise works its mental magic" (Holmes 2022). My wife and I have spent a combined fifty-five years and counting knowing the benefits of exercise, and yet the point to what we are addressing in this book is that corruptive practices by so-called intelligent people with degrees have done the very opposite for our children. This article is very correct, but the corruptive nature in education and fitness specifically has not allowed or figured out how to make this a daily experience for people. Again it is our hope that this book becomes the blueprint of all these concepts because it really does comes down to what I learned back in Coach Stucky's weight room and the idea of actual proper training without the snake oil, and physical education for all kids every day in public schools is what is necessary. Teaching, curriculum, and public education need a complete overhaul (i.e., nothing public education is doing currently is appropriate, so until that overhaul happens, the same rehash of old trash will continue, and the only thing that is actually new is that they just put a new name to a wrong echo chamber to follow and call it change)!

"Exercise, they are learning, has profound effects on the brain's structure itself, and it also provides other, more subtle benefits such as focus, a sense of accomplishment, and sometimes social stimulation—all of which are therapeutic in their own right. And while more is generally better, even modest levels of physical activity, such as a daily walk, can pay big dividends for mental health" (Holmes 2022). This is just a simple example of why our academic interventions were so popular with the kids, but that was unique to us and our circumstance because the public schools and all its complexities are doing so many inappropriate practices in all aspects that it becomes just a Band-Aid on a wound that won't heal.

"It's very potent intervention to be physically active," said Anders Hovland, a clinical psychologist at the University of Bergen in Norway. "But that knowledge has barely begun to percolate into practice," said Joseph Firth, a mental health researcher at the University of Manchester in the United Kingdom. "Just ask a hundred people receiving mental health care how many are getting exercise prescriptions as part of that care. You wouldn't find many," Firth said (Holmes 2022). This is exactly true! We are sure that the force 46 concept of physical education and fitness training is the answer to dangerous train wrecks that have and will continue to occur. Hopefully, this book becomes the transformational knowledge that completely overhauls all the entities and issues addressed in this book and actually leads to immediate change and benefit for all.

The importance of PE class at all levels on a daily basis should be clear, but I would like to discuss elementary school in particular. The highlight of our kids' day is when they have PE. Many can hardly control themselves because they are so excited. At the elementary school, in particular, some type of game play is vitally important. How the new PE could sit there and promote the use of pedometers for walking kids and running on expensive machines versus small group games with and without competition is truly the scam of the century next to some of the previously addressed issues (e.g., plyometrics, Western periodization, FitGram testing, etc.). We can't list everything we created in our program, but we will attempt to give the basic elementary class structure and grading during the forty-minute elementary PE class. What we have to get across is that fitness centers, heart rate monitors, pedometers, bike riding, snowshoeing, invalid and inappropriate fitness testing and then self-promotion *is not great physical education*. Game play—both structured and unstructured, both small groups and team—is absolutely essential for full development and health of our children, and PE should be offered to every child every day. The grading system becomes very relevant to this, and that is why we applied the factors of fitness to be the model grading scale.

The definitions of the factors of fitness come from Siff 2003. The brief examples as well as the description of motor planning and static and dynamic balance are from our program.

S-Factors and Grading System

Throughout my twenty-five years of teaching high-level physical education, I have been able to observe many issues in the educational system. Government mandates, political agendas, self-promotion, unions, and school boards are all involved in a complex system where everyone is considered equal and all opinions are given credence even with the shared statement that everyone is doing what is in the best interest of the children. Having watched all these complex interplay for over twenty-five years, I decided to take the lead to change grading once and for all for elementary physical education and try and insure that if vertically aligned as it should be, the new grading scale would definitely lend itself to the importance of physical education and actually allow for students' understanding of what fitness is and how to maintain high fitness for the rest of their lives.

The book *Supertraining* is one of the very best books ever written. It is scientifically written by two of the world's foremost authorities on fitness and training. Dr. Mel Siff and Dr. Yuri Verkhoshansky, by the sixth edition of the book, really gave us the scientific basis to solve many problems. However, 99 percent of my colleagues over the years had never even heard of this book. Simply put, over the years, most of the colleges and universities spent their time teaching the cardiovascular doctrine (as stated earlier) that has caused physical education and fitness in the United States to be set back sixty years and counting.

I researched the S-factors section many times over the years and finally decided to do something big and make those factors be what kids should be graded on. If children understood these factors of fitness, then they would likely have the knowledge to maintain a fit lifestyle for the entirety of their lives. This is always the said goal of many state and federal mandates, yet the result never happens and this, in turn, has led to many self-promoters and corrupt officials laying claim to be experts. The factors of fitness scale is a game changer for physical education programs, and it can lead to great physical education class structure that my wife and I already have created and performed for many years.

The S-factors, as Siff and Verkhoshansky wrote, are as follows: strength, speed, suppleness, stamina (general endurance/local muscular endurance), skill (neuromuscular efficiency), structure (somatotype, size, and shape), and spirit (psychological preparedness).

Within the scope of skill, there is also a fitness quality known as style (individual manner of expressing a particular skill).

The following are the fitness factors simply defined for the elementary physical education program:

> Spirit (psychological factors)
> Motivation to achieve certain goals
> Aggression (desire to succeed/desire to compete against themselves or with others appropriately)
> Concentration
> Focus
> Attention
> Ability to tolerate pain or working discomfort while sustaining effort
> Ability to cope with stress or anxiety
> Attitude
> Mood state
> Personality

Alertness and vigilance
Ability to manage distractions
Ability to relax effectively

Relative strength-ability to hold or move body weight appropriately with little difficulty.

Static relative strength-ability to hold the body in proper position for time (e.g., static push-up, static squat, plank, etc.).

Dynamic relative strength-ability to move body (e.g., push-up, bodyweight squat, walking single-leg squat, bear walk, frog jump, etc.).

Flexibility (suppleness)-range of movement (ROM) of a specific joint with respect to a particular degree of freedom.

Static passive flexibility-stationary stretching (seated foot to knee, butterfly, legs apart, reverse seal, etc.).

Dynamic active flexibility-combined strength and stretching exercises (walking lung, walking single-leg squat, inch worm, high knee carioca, etc.).

Speed-ability of muscles to produce movement rapidly.

Speed strength-ability to quickly execute an unloaded movement or a movement against a relatively small external resistance.

Quickness-ability of the central nervous system to contract, relax, or control muscle function without involvement of any preliminary stretch. (Reaction time between stimulus and response [e.g., partner tennis ball off wall].)

Reactive ability-neuromuscular ability to generate explosive force requiring a preliminary stretch and rapidity of reaction (e.g., three hop)

Skill

Neuromuscular efficiency-the skill with which one executes a given movement and relates to how efficiently and intensively one recruits muscle fibers in the appropriate muscle groups to produce the movement pattern accurately and powerfully (e.g., dot drills, two foot agility hoop hop, icky shuffle, scissor switch, etc.).

Visual motor control-tracking, hand-eye coordination (wall toss and catch, wall throw and catch, throw and catch with a partner, basketball dribble, etc.).

Endurance (Stamina)

General endurance-in terms of the cardiovascular-respiratory functions that provide the necessary oxygen and the appropriate state of the neuromuscular system (sixty-second jog, ninety-second interval jog, two-minute jog, etc.).

Local muscular endurance-endurance is associated more with enhancing the ability of the muscles to utilize a higher percentage of the oxygen already in the blood than with increasing the amount of oxygen in the bloodstream and improving the oxygen supply to the working muscles (rope slam, sprint relay, floor hockey, zone ball, corner soccer basketball, etc.).

Motor planning-ability to conceive, plan, and carry out a skilled nonhabitual motor act in the correct sequence from beginning to end (e.g., dot drills, speed ladder drills, agility hoop drills, etc.).

Static and Dynamic Balance

Static balance-ability to stay upright or stay in control of body movement, coordination, and maintaining equilibrium when stationary (e.g., static squat, static push-up, dome cones, etc.).

Dynamic balance-maintaining equilibrium while moving. Coordination is the ability to move two or more body parts under control smoothly and efficiently (e.g., single-leg squats, bodyweight squats, standing knee lift, top claw, balance beam with objects, various jumps and lands, frog jump, lateral bounding, etc.).

The grading scale I developed from this documented science is as follows:

1) Spirit (psychological factors)
   Motivations to achieve certain goals; desire
       to succeed and compete/vigilance
   Concentration/attention/focus/alertness
   Attitude/mood state/personality
   Ability to manage distractions/ability to
       relax effectively

2) Strength
   A. Static relative strength
      Technique
      Ability
      Effort
   B. Dynamic relative strength
      Technique
      Ability
      Effort

3) Flexibility
   A. Static passive flexibility
      Technique
      Ability
      Effort
   B. Dynamic active flexibility
      Technique
      Ability
      Effort

4) Speed
   A. Speed strength
      Technique
      Ability
      Effort

B. Quickness
Technique
Ability
Effort
C. Reactive ability
Technique
Ability
Effort

5) Skill
A. Neuromuscular efficiency
Technique
Ability
Effort
B. Visual motor control
Technique
Ability
Effort

6) Stamina
A. General endurance
Technique
Ability
Effort
B. Local muscular endurance
Technique
Ability
Effort

7) Motor planning
Technique
Ability
Effort

8) Static and Dynamic balance
   A. Static balance
      Technique
      Ability
      Effort

Look at categorizing honors physical education or advanced physical education and general physical education.

The scale for points is as follows:

> one point-does not demonstrate the standard technique/ability/effort
> two points-demonstrates standard technique but not standard ability/effort
> three points-demonstrates standard technique and ability and effort
> four points-demonstrates above standard technique and ability

We believe the new grading system will help parents and students understand the fitness factors that make a well-rounded human being. Unfortunately, human fitness has been improperly thought of for many years. This is mainly due to misrepresentation of various fitness models and concepts that have been publicized by self-serving interests, personal agendas, and proprietary programming. The fact is there are many elements to human fitness, and they all have relevance and importance. The goal for physical education in schools is to teach the definition of fitness by emphasizing all fitness factors along with activities and movement patterns for each one. By introducing these fitness factors in elementary school, it will allow us to identify strengths and weaknesses in these initial fitness factors to help the children make improvements in necessary categories. As the students progress through the K-5 physical education curriculum, the categories should expand through middle school and high school (e.g., speed strength, absolute strength, explosive strength, etc.). This will allow every student to graduate with an actual understanding of what fitness is and how to improve throughout their lifetime.

It is important to realize that the grades in each fitness factor will go up or down as the students demonstrate their individual ability throughout the year and future years. Society has changed drastically as outlined in the new PE chapter. Most of the kids in our area do not participate in much activity on a daily basis. Many of the sport programs are more about participation that has created kids who are still out of shape and obese, but at least, they participate in something. This is not acceptable, and we believe this grading system, and philosophy is what can help get the real importance and need for daily physical education in public schools and available to all students and not be under the failed cardiovascular doctrine echo chamber or circle jerk—whichever you prefer to use!

We developed the above grading and philosophy for grades K-4 through fifth grade. Obviously then, the curriculum should vertically align and increase through the middle and high school. This would ensure that children actually can graduate with the real knowledge of fitness and be free from the differing echo chambers of the past sixty years and counting as described in the first chapter.

The grading scale would then increase its categories vertically by adding the following: absolute strength, speed strength, and explosive strength.

Categorization of strength capabilities into these four types can be somewhat restrictive because all of them are interrelated in their production and development despite their inherent specificity. They are rarely, if ever, displayed separately but are the components of every movement. The strength ability most characteristic of sporting activities is explosive strength, as displayed in acyclic and cyclic movements. Acyclic movements are distinguished by brief episodes of powerful muscular work and cyclic movements by the maintenance of optimal power for a relatively long time. If attention is paid to the fact that the explosive character with which strength is displayed is determined by the presence of absolute strength or speed-strength (depending upon external conditions), then two general abilities, namely explosive strength and strength-endurance, are the basis for the production of all sporting movements. (Siff 2003)

Since the essence of sport is human movement, and a societal need and goal for humans is to maintain the ability to move and be fit over an individual's lifetime, then, clearly, this information should be inherent to a physical education program. The cardiovascular doctrine ignored it. The new PE chose to not cater to athletes, and in short, the train wreck has easily continued since 1965 minimally.

One of our goals with physical education is that after graduation, kids will have the intrinsic desire and physical movement ability (whether a nonathlete or athlete) to be able to play vigorously and train vigorously throughout their life! We have observed in our almost sixty years of teaching many thousands of children that many of our teenagers do not move or control their bodies appropriately because of promoted knowledge like the cardiovascular doctrine, poor research-driven information, and proprietary programming for self-promotion presented in this book. Therefore, many kids are already on the path of leading sedentary lives, and it only gets progressively worse as the kids get to the end of their twenties. Much of our population is not capable of playing racquetball, or basketball or adult hockey or anything that is vigorous. This has been enabled by the echo chambers of false knowledge that only athletes are strong, walking ten thousand steps a day will make you fit, girls shouldn't lift because they will get big, walk on a treadmill and talk to your best friend, or watch TV, and that is a vigorous workout. BMI is the holy grail of informing people they are fat even though it does not address lean muscle. All these has led to physical education not being important in the minds of much of society and the fact that many physical education programs are implemented very poorly at best.

Within the higher level grading scale then two additional terms should be involved in a great physical education program. "Starting-strength and acceleration-strength. Starting-strength is the ability to quickly develop the greatest possible force at the initial moment of tension. Acceleration-strength is the ability to build up a working force as rapidly as possible once the contraction has begun" (Siff 2003). This factual science is what actually can help a physical educator create their activities appropriately. Smart physical education has most, if not all, of these elements in the daily class. Smart physical education does not run long boring units like pedometer walking for forty minutes three times a week and then arrogantly preach that they are teaching kids to be physically active or somehow are going to fitness test students and are making a positive impact in their lives. This would be the time in the vertical alignment of physical education to add the idea of strength and fitness.

The correct scientific terms of work capacity, fitness, and preparedness are extremely important to teach and have all students actually know what each term means and what it feels like to develop these related factors. "Work capacity refers to the general ability of the body as a machine to produce work of different intensity and duration using the appropriate energy systems of the body. Fitness refers to the specific ability to use this work capacity to execute a given task under particular conditions. In general terms, fitness may be defined as the ability to cope with the demands of a specific task efficiently and safely. Preparedness, unlike fitness, is not stable but varies with time. It comprises two components, one that is slow changing and the other that is fast changing" (Siff 2003).

The slow component is fitness, and the fast component is exercise-induced fatigue. Although the concept of fitness would seem to be intuitively obvious and well-accepted, one should note this distinction between fitness and preparedness. The term physical fitness refers to the functional state of the slow-changing physiological components relating to motor activity. One's fitness state does not vary significantly over any period up to as much as several days in length.

However, one's ability to express fitness at any instant may be substantially affected positively or negatively by mental state, sickness, fatigue, sleepiness, and other fairly transient factors. This ability, or instantaneous preparedness, is defined at any given instant and varies from moment to moment. Training or conditioning is the process whereby body and mind are prepared to reach a certain level of work capacity and fitness (Siff 2003).

While it can be deemed appropriate to then have kids on a treadmill, we do not agree for the most part. Teaching kids with strength and conditioning concepts (multi-joint free weights) and vigorous play and movement skill is clearly our statement on this. Most physical education or school educators do not have any knowledge of the books we are citing in our book. We also have found that even when an individual comes across cited information, their perceptions somehow skew the intended purpose, and things become a mess quickly. That mess becomes fact, and the process keeps repeating itself.

Many of the concepts from specialization come from this kind of cited information. When intelligent individuals see that certain fitness factors are more important than others in a certain sport or circumstance, then philosophies and paradigms are developed, and the track coach wants his/her athletes to not lift because the coach believes that lifting makes you slow, and VO^2 uptake is how a runner gets better. Or a swimmer should not lift because they might get bulky or big. It becomes even more complex because what if the kids are multisport, and the swimmer also plays football, and the football coach wants to train a certain way and then when the player goes into swimming season, the swimming coach wants to train a different way. This is how the train wreck happens, and the kids invariably do not ever reach their potential. All the while, the training programs from the coaches are often done by people who just love their sport. These coaches are not even close to being strength and conditioning coaches with any true experience or academic background. We have seen many times that these same coaches find physical education class as unimportant and foster the same myths we have been addressing throughout our book.

Classroom Design

All the previous source of information and personal experience led us to develop the K-5 physical education program specifically. We then developed how to align the program through K-12 vertically, which, to date, nobody has. The three parts of the force 46 physical education program are early movement, strength/agility/skill, and play or activity. For elementary students, it is always play. For middle and high school students, it would be play as well as free weightlifting or other physical activities.

I had the opportunity to move back to the elementary level after teaching for fifteen years at the high school level. I had been a part of developing a highly recognized physical education program in the United States. I was very much against how the recognition and notoriety was developed as well as against some of the philosophical teaching that some of my colleagues presented to students (i.e., following the cardiovascular doctrine). However, I was able to implement all the parts of great physical education that I felt were mandatory, and the rest is history. Moving to the elementary school allowed me to develop a physical education program that I felt could be groundbreaking. It was our belief that our elementary physical education programs should model for what elementary physical education should be for our children to engage in.

The first thing I did was reach out to Todd Burkey. Todd was part of my national strength and conditioning group of friends, and we spoke at many strength and conditioning conferences over the years. Todd worked at the Cleveland Clinic before becoming a head athletic trainer and also head strength and conditioning coach over many years at Youngstown State University. Todd currently trained the Chinese women's Olympic hockey team and is back in China to coach the Olympic basketball teams as well. Many of my colleagues stated that Todd was way beyond, knowledge wise, than most minds in the United States when it came to training and injury prevention. I definitely agree with that statement. I asked Todd, "What do you think is the single most important aspect missing in elementary physical education today?"

Todd immediately said, "Early movement!"

I immediately made early movement a daily priority in my physical education plan. The following aspects became a daily part of my elementary physical education program: I typically started my elementary class with a warm-up jog, interval jog, or if I wanted the kids to be stationary in their movement spots, then we did jumping jacks, jog in place, and rebound jumps to get the body ready to exercise. The movement spots mean that each student had a specific spot to stand at. I used the lines on the gym floor to create five or six movement lines with five or six movement spots for each line. This allowed for great spacing in the gym for the early movement and joint mobility drills. Many of my joint mobility drills came from reading Pavel Tsatsouline's *Super Joints: Russian Longevity Secrets for Pain-Free Movement, Maximum Mobility, and Flexible Strength* and *Relax into Stretch: Instant Flexibility through Mastering Muscle Tension* books. We also emphasized relative strength and flexibility exercises at the movement spots. After the warm-up and joint mobility portion of class, which can be approximately eight to twelve minutes, I would have the students walk their movement lines back to the end of the gym to start the dynamic early movement part of class.

The dynamic movement part of class consisted of relative strength body movements that addressed the fitness factors described earlier. I created movement drills for first and second grade and then created higher-level movement drills for third through fifth grade. There obviously is some overlap in drills between the grades. Some of the basic movement drills for first and second grade were skip, gallop, shuffle, back pedal, frog jump and jog, three hop and jog, crossover jog, sprint relay, etc. Some of the basic movement drills for third through fifth grade were ham kicks, walking singleleg squats, carioca, tapioca, high knee carioca, sprint relay, etc.

After both aspects of the early movement portion of class, the second part of our elementary class was the strength/agility and skill stations. This concept mirrors what my wife had successfully implemented in our early childhood learning center (grades K-4 and K-5). The list is infinite of the activities that we performed in this section. I was able to get a climbing cargo net as I developed the program as well as getting rope slams and sandbag kettlebells as well as an endless list of fun things over time, so our stations were really incredible looking back. Little to none of the equipment I put together over the nine years was there when I came. I was able to implement this philosophy with little equipment, and the kids loved it! Each year, I kept getting more and more equipment on about a thousand dollar budget; and by the time I was in year five, I had what I would consider the best elementary physical education program and set up in the country. I am most proud that it was built with no grant money or any specialized help. When conceptualizing how to develop a great daily physical education experience, the science of direct and indirect connections becomes very important. This is very important in both strength and conditioning and physical education program design.

> Direct connection is characterized by a relationship between two abilities (general and partial, essential and nonessential, positive and negative connections).
>
> Indirect connection is also a relation when there is an essential, direct connection between two abilities (e.g., there is no correlation between abilities A and B in the figure below, but they are nevertheless connected through the third ability). (Siff 2003)

The latter connection is the most characteristic structure of physical fitness. For example, there is no direct, significant connection between running speed and a sprinter's absolute leg strength (it has already been mentioned that this connection is negative at the partial level). However, there is close connection with jumping exercises that are also rather closely connected with running speed. This emphasizes how important it is to have a clear representation of the structure of an athlete's special strength fitness and use this to determine tasks and provide means of special strength training.

The indirect connections between motor abilities can be more complex. Thus, there is no direct, significant connection between the height achieved in a vertical jump and the absolute strength of the legs. However, absolute strength determines the magnitude of the maximal force of the take-off (fmax), which, in turn, influences the magnitude of the impulse (f.t) of the push off and, ultimately, the height of the jump. (*Supertraining Sixth Edition*, 117 and 204)

The third and final part of class was play. My wife and I believe that play is essential and should be promoted every day for elementary students at a minimum. We have seen over the years that the new PE was pushing the cardiovascular doctrine and expensive machines, heart rate monitors, and pedometers. These types of devices are all tied to the proprietary programs and fitness fads. If you ever had the chance to watch our kids go through a forty-minute class in all three phases of our class structure, then you would not have to ask why we did not waste the time or money on these technologies.

Importance of Early Movement

The following information my wife and I added within our belief system many years ago comes from the book *Movement with a Purpose: Perceptual Motor-Lesson Plans for Young Children* written by Madeleine Brehm and Nancy T. Tindell. This is a book that is more relevant now than when they published it in 1983! In *Movement with a Purpose: Perceptual Motor-Lesson Plans for Young Children*, to develop self-esteem, we need to develop a student who delights in and takes confidence in moving his or her body and a student who is at home in that body. The aim of movement with a purpose is to develop purposeful, joyful, and creative movement to prepare children for a lifetime of healthy activity. The authors went on to state that persons with reading problems can hear the news on TV, and persons who dislike math can use the calculator to balance the checkbook, but people with poorly developed motor skills have a hard time circumventing the problem!

All through our lives, we need to move our bodies through space in an efficient, effective manner. A truly complete program of movement is one that sets time aside for structured and sequentially developed activities for children. This is not to take away from the importance of free play or recess either! The authors went on to state that teachers and parents cannot easily detect poor coordination on a balance beam while a child is running around the playground. Spotting a student's inability to distinguish right from left is easily missed during free play. Often, running and skipping are the basic locomotor skills observed on the playground, but we want to look further to see if the child can jump, slide, and hop. Can the child hop on the left and the right foot? If so, is the hip a smooth and coordinated action? When bouncing a ball, does the child demonstrate proper bouncing methods? Can the child keep his or her eyes on the ball to catch successfully? All these areas, along with many others, can be addressed with the authors' ideas as well as in force 46 class design.

These things should be every day in great physical education. Great physical education does not entail just exposing the kids to something and then moving on. It should be a philosophy and clearly is a much needed one. The proprietary programming of the past and current physical education supports do not do this. They just push the next magic bullet, the next pricey machine or technology (e.g., treadmills and pedometers), and pass it off as great PE. This is a scam that never changes. Hopefully, this book and the great information in it will be the one to put finality to the question, What is great physical education and why it should be provided every day to every child?

Siff 2003 states that athletic performance may be described in terms of a complex interaction of many movements so that the fundamental phenomenon underlying all sports tasks is human movement. This statement alone says that the new PE nonsense and cardiovascular doctrine is 100 percent completely false, and the narrative has been destructive to the importance of physical education. The new PE actually performed reverse discrimination against athletes as well as confusing their own favorite saying "we don't want to just roll out the ball and not teach." Just rolling out the ball and standing there is exactly what the new PE accomplished with the heart rate monitors, fixed machine centers, and following the cardiovascular doctrine, standing there and watching kids inefficiently work for forty minutes and shouting a few words of encouragement and then checking their watches at the end to see if they deserve a good grade! Or my other favorite is give all students a pedometer and watch them walk for forty minutes and then see how many steps they get. If any human being thinks that that is teaching, then this book is not for you!

Continuing with the movement with a purpose idea, Siff and Verkhoshansky stated that absolute strength, explosive strength, speed strength, and strength endurance are inherent in all human movement, and they are rarely, if ever, displayed separately. Sport then becomes a problem-solving activity in which movements are used to produce the necessary solutions. This is very true, and you would think that the so-called academic people and state and federal government experts (we use that term loosely) would understand then the importance of physical education and learning for our children. Yet many so-called academic or great schools cut physical education and exercise out of the school day because we somehow need all children to pass irrelevant state tests on algebra, science, and English. None of this is even remotely academic or intelligent to me. The nonsense that is going on in education today is a shame, and we feel it very important to say something to correct the situation because if we do not, then the last sixty years of experience in education for my wife and I will be sad!

References

Books:

Hackenschmidt, G. 1908. *The Way to Live: In Health and Physical Fitness.*

Kubik, B. D. 1996. *Dinosaur Training: Lost Secrets of Strength and Development.* Brooks D. Kubik.

Siff, M. C. 2003. *Facts and Fallacies of Fitness.* Printed in Denver ISBN 1-868-183-8.

Tsatsouline, P. 2001. *The Russian Kettlebell Challenge: Xtreme Fitness for Hard Living Comrades.* Dragon Door Publications, Inc.

Zatsiorsky, V. M. 1995. *Science and Practice of Strength Training.* Human Kinetics.

Siff, M. C. 2003. *Supertraining 6th Edition.* Supertraining Institute, Denver, USA.

Brehm, M. and Tindell, N. T. 1983. *Movement with a Purpose: Perceptual Motor-Lesson Plans for Young Children.* Parker Publishing Company, Inc., West Nyack, New York.

(1987) *1984 Weightlifting Yearbook*. Translated by Andrew Charniga Jr. Livonia, Michigan: Sportivny Press, 1987.

Online Sources:

Appleby, J. 2022. "BMI: The Mismeasure of Weight and the Mistreatment of Obesity."
https://khn.org/news/article/bmi-obesity-treatment-prescription-weight-loss-drugs-vegovy-insurance-coverage/

Hudson, R. W. 2022. "8 Outstanding Benefits of the Barbell Back Squat."
https://www.boxrox.com/benefits-of-the-barbell-back-squat/

Richardson, B. 2022. "The Best Workout Routine Ever, According to Science."
https://www.wellness52.com/best-workout-routine/

Loewe, E. 2022. "Yet *Another* Study Finds that Regular Resistance Training Builds Muscle Strength."
https://www.mindbodygreen.com/articles/resistance-training-over-high-intensity-study

Nelson, J. Q. 2022. "We Need to Be Supporting Our Teachers." *Fox News*.
https//mail.google.com/mail/u/3/?ik=304d887e92&view=pt&search=all&permthid=thread-f%3A1743034697200022640&simpl=msg-f%3A1743034697…

Heffernan, A. 2022. "How Functional Bodybuilding Is Designed to Be Kinder to Your Body."
https://www.menshealth.com/fitness/a40880755/marcus-filly-functional-bodybuilding/

Olson, A. 2022. "Nick Saban Confirms Alabama Is Providing Academic Bonus Payments After UA Left Out of ESPN Report." https://www.saturdaydownsouth.com.

2022. "5 Incredible Ways Exercise Improves Brain Function." https://scitechdaily.com/5-incredible-ways-exercise-im-proves-brain-function/

Burdman, P. 2022. "To Keep Students in STEM fields, Let's Weed Out the Weed-Out Math Classes." Scientific American, A Division of Springer Nature America, Inc. https://www.scientificamerican.com/article/to-keep-students-in-stem-fields-lets-weed-out-the-weed-out-math-classes/

McMurtrie, B. 2022. "A Stunning Level of Student Disconnection." The Chronicle of Higher Education. https://www.chronicle.com/article/a-stunning-level-of-stu-dent-disconnection?utm_source=Iterable&utm_medium=e-mail&utm_campaign=campaign_5765417_nl_Academe-Today_date_20221219&cid=at&source=&sourceid=&cid2=-gen_login_refresh

Hughes, A. 2022. "HIIT vs Weight Training: Which Will Make You Fitter, A Physiotherapist Explains the Difference." https://www.sciencefocus.com/the-human-body/hiit-vs-weight-training-which-will-make-you-fitter-a-physiotherapist-explains-the-difference/

Grandin, T. 2022. "Against Algebra." https://www.theatlantic.com/ideas/archive/2022/10/against algebra/671643/

James, L. 2022. "Strength Testing and Training: Understanding Which Strength Quality to Focus on." https://www.sportsmith.co/articles/testing-and-training-ath-lete-strength/

Holmes, B. 2022. "Exercise Boosts the Brain—and Mental Health." *The Washington Post.* https://www.washingtonpost.com/health/2022/02/19/exercise-mental-health/

Harrison, M. 2022. "Scientists Find that Lifting Weights Offers No Benefit Over Simply Lowering Them." https://futurism.com/neoscope/lifting-weights-no-benefit-simply-lowering.

Anderer, J. 2022. "Strength Training Key to Long Life? Weak Muscles 'Could Be the New Smoking' When It Comes to Healthy Aging." *Study Finds.* https://studyfinds.org/strength-training-weak-muscles-healthy-aging/.

Karthik, Krishnan. 2020. "Our Education System Is Losing Relevance. Here's How to Unleash Its Potential." World Economic Forum. www.weforum.org/agenda/2020/04/our-education-system-is-losing-relevance-heres-how-to-update-it/

Low, Chris. "Clemson Tigers Coach Dabo Swinney Says There Needs to Be "Complete Blowup" of College Football." https://www.espn.ph/college-football/story/_/id/33700813/clemson-tigers-coach-dabo-swinney-says-there-needs-complete-blowup-college football. Accessed April 8, 2022.

Murphy, Tom. 2022. "Barry Foster a Key Cog in Hatfield's Flexbone Offense." Arkansas Democrat Gazette. https://www.arkansasonline.com/news/2022/apr/01/barry-foster-a-key-cog-in-hatfields-flexbone/.

Farkas, Dan. 2007. "John Stucky Has Died." www.volnation.com>-forum>threads. April 13, 2007.

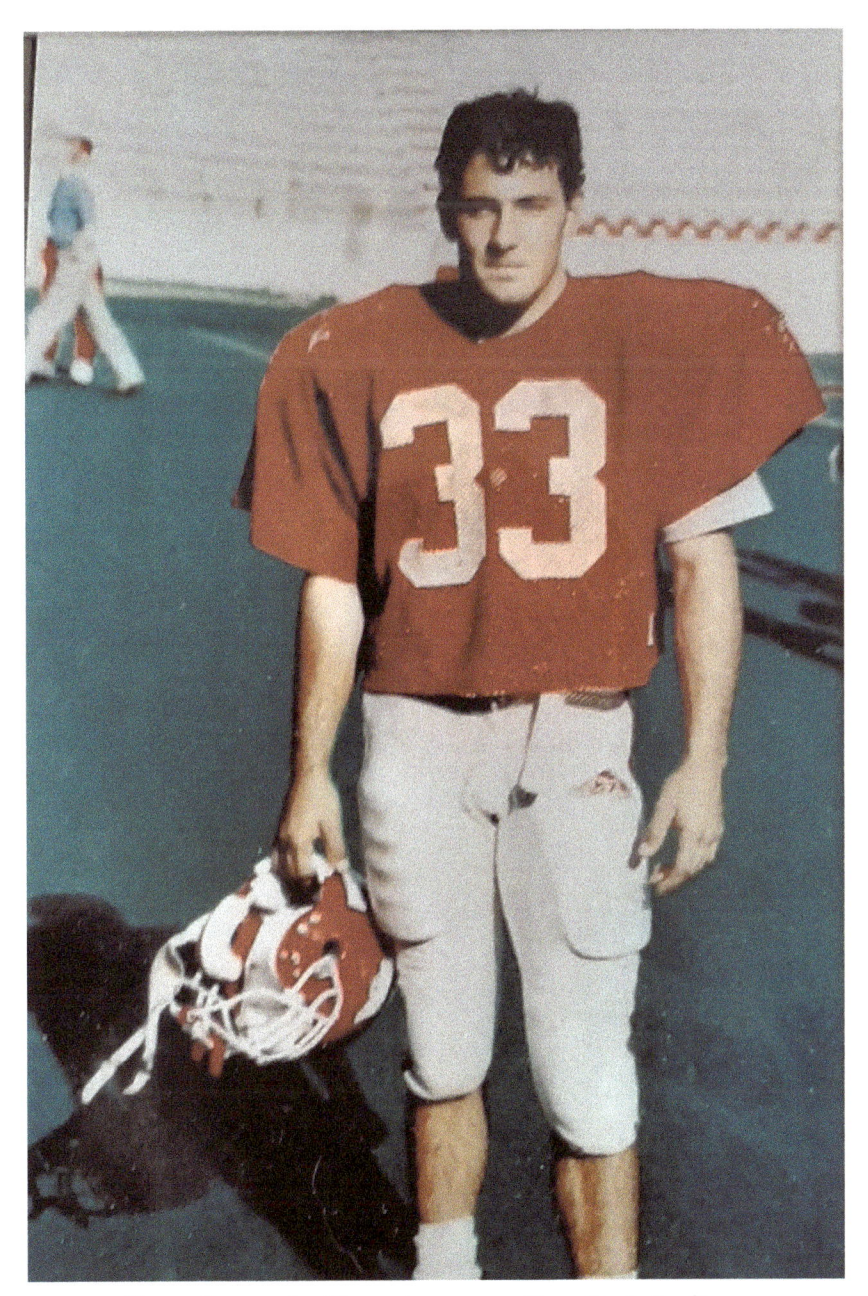

Tony after a red-white scrimmage at Razorback Stadium.

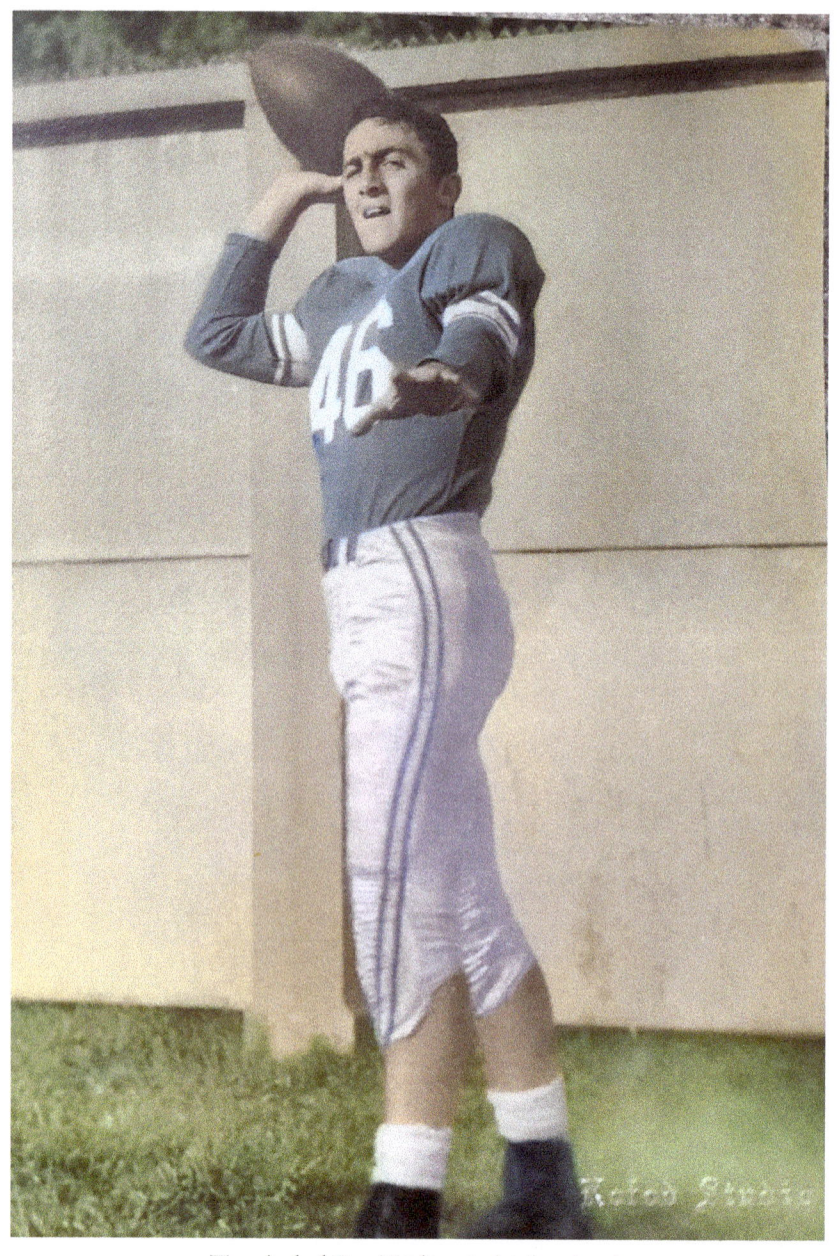

Tony's dad Jim Tridico in high school

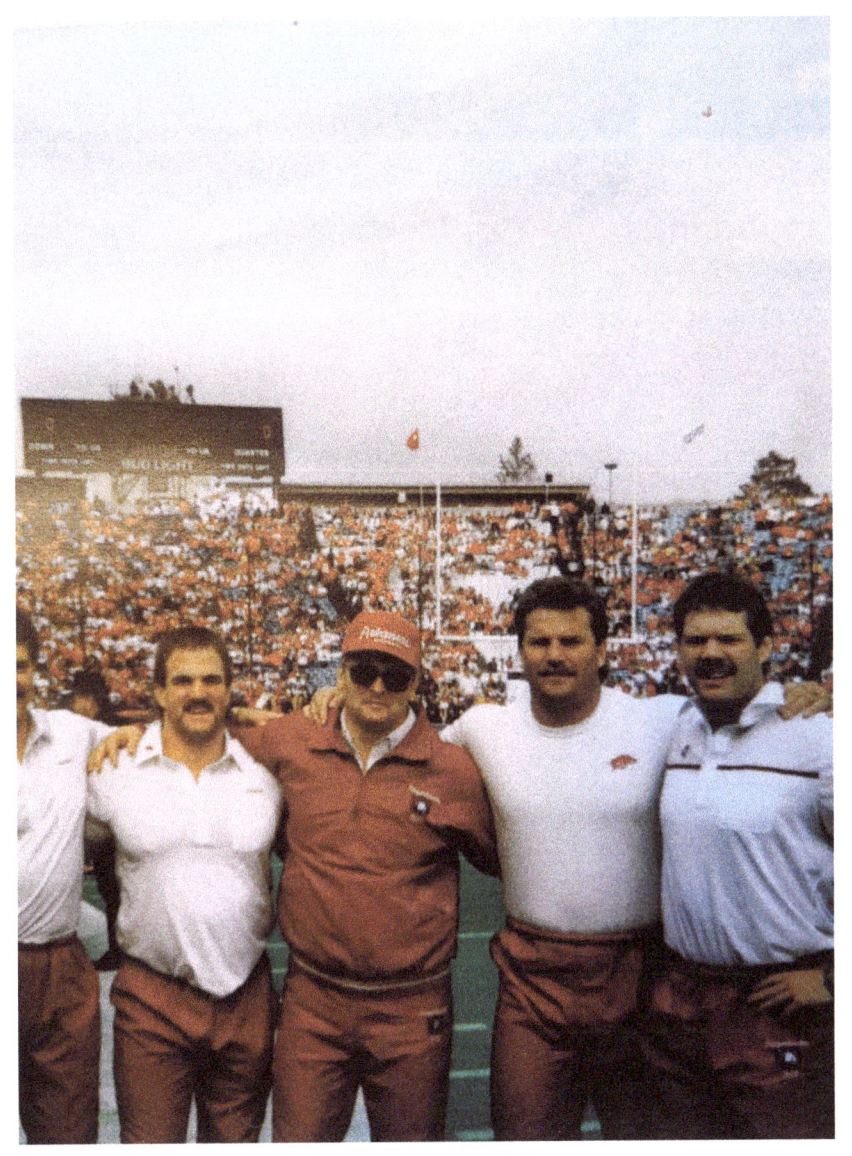

Coach Stucky (middle)

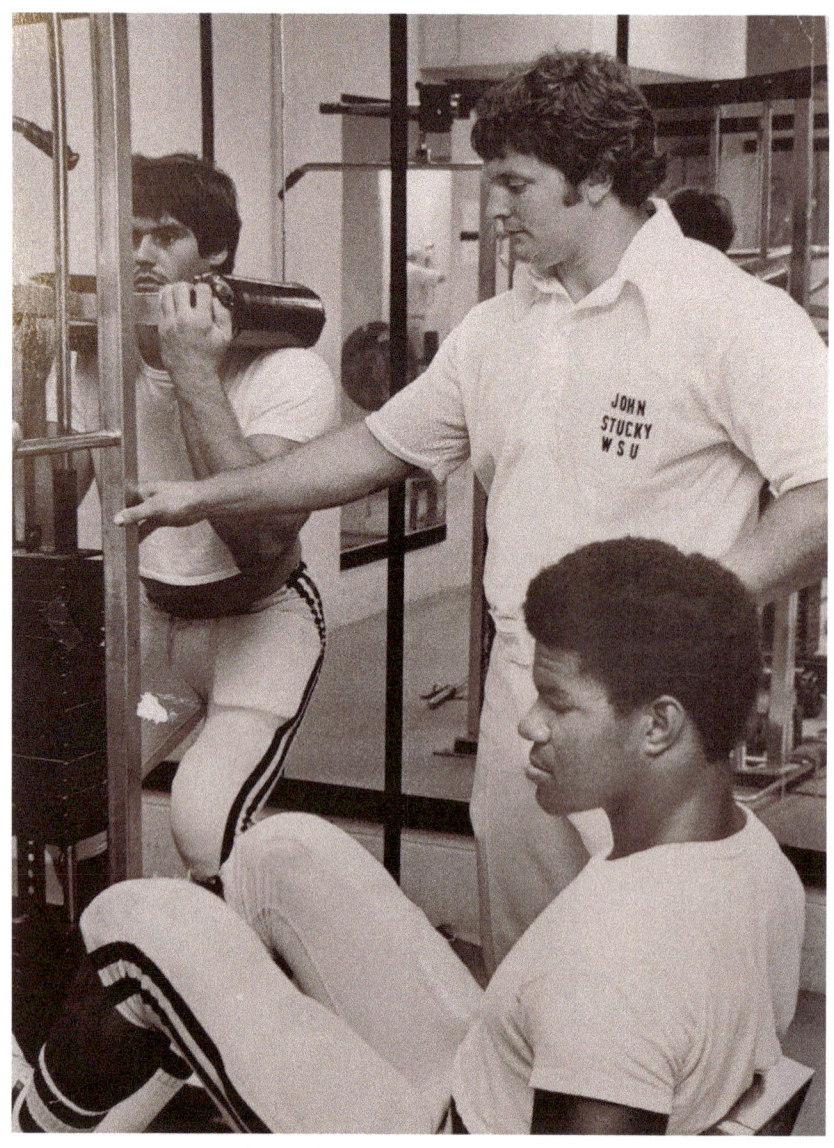

Coach Stucky at Wichita State University

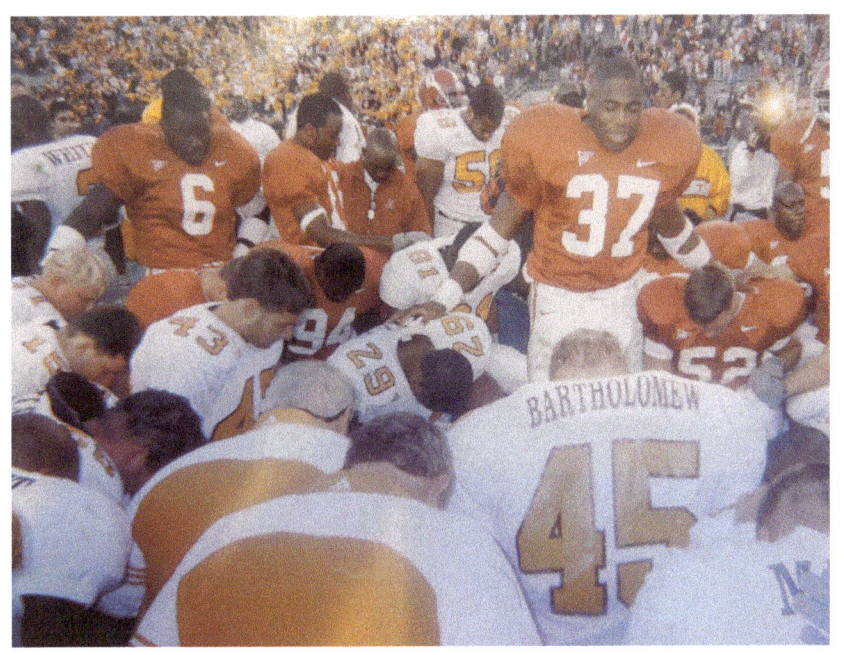

Coach Stucky kneeling in prayer after the 1998 National
Championship game with players from both teams
(this picture defines who Coach Stucky was)

About the Author

Tony trained as a football player under head strength and conditioning coach, John Stucky, who was named one of the ten master strength and conditioning coaches by the CSCCA. The award is the highest honor that can be achieved as a strength and conditioning coach. Tony was a two-term national strength and conditioning association Pennsylvania state director, and he was a certified strength and conditioning specialist (CSCS) for many years. Tony has over thirty years of experience writing training programs for all levels and goals. He also earned a top five finalist recognition for the NSCA national high school strength and conditioning coach of the year award. Tony annually presented at and held state level strength and conditioning clinics for fourteen years and continues to present when available.

Tony was an assistant strength and conditioning coach under the direction of Joe Kenn at Boise State University and participated in coaching twenty-seven division I sports teams, both men and women. He also competed on the Boise State University powerlifting team. Tony won first place bench press in the beast of the northeast powerlifting competition 1989. He also won first place in the bench press at the Idaho state championships in 1996 and first place bench press and overall best lifter at the house power bench press extravaganza in Bosie, Idaho, 1997. Tony was a University of Arkansas football player for three years in the early 1990s. He also earned the head football coach position for the Pennsylvania big 30 all-star game in 2010.

Tony graduated from the University of Arkansas with a bachelor's of science degree in kinesiology. He completed all his graduate-level classes in the master's of science in exercise and sport studies at Boise State University. He also graduated with a master's in educational leadership (principal certified K-12) from Edinboro University. Tony is a twenty-five-year veteran physical education teacher and coach. He created a comprehensive elementary school physical education program curriculum and design and grading system. Tony earned and was recognized as a Golden Apple Award-Winning Teacher for the 2020–2021 school year at Pleasantville Elementary School in Pleasantville, Pennsylvania.

Tony retired from teaching early to follow his passion to start a strength and conditioning business called Force 46 Strength and Conditioning LLC. He currently trains a wide range of clients ages eight to seventy-two. This book is a special tribute and thank you to Coach Stucky and a special thanks to Coach's wife, Jeanne, and his son, Phillip. Also, a special thanks to my parents James and Joan Tridico, my son James, and my wife Jenny for her input for the physical education chapters.